COPING

WITH

FIBROMYALGIA

by

Othniel J. Seiden, MD
& Jane L. Bilett, PhD

Cover Art
by Capri Brock

A Books To Believe In Publication
All Rights Reserved
Copyright 2009 by Othniel Seiden & Jane L. Bilett

Proudly Published in the USA by

Boomer Book Series

ISBN: 1519438311

DEDICATIONS

**To Dr. David Wiener
& the Orthopedic Department of
Kaiser Permanente - for replacing
both of my arthritic hips...**

TABLE OF CONTENTS

Chapter 1

What is Fibromyalgia?

Fibromyalgia is a chronic arthritic condition characterized by widespread aching and pain in the muscles, ligaments and tendons and multiple joints, and is accompanied by debilitating fatigue and multiple tender points on the body where even the slightest pressure may cause pain. Fibromyalgia is more common in women than in men. The intensity of symptoms may vary from time to time, but they will probably never disappear completely. However, Fibromyalgia is not progressive nor is it life threatening.

The Risk Factors for Fibromyalgia

Fibromyalgia occurs more often in women than in men and tends to develop during early and middle adulthood, but it has on rare occasion occurred in children as well as in older adults. Fibromyalgia is estimated to affect 2–4% of the population, with a female to male incidence ratio of approximately 10 to 1. It is unclear whether sleeping difficulties are a cause or the result of Fibromyalgia, but it appears that people with sleep disorders, like nighttime muscle spasms in their legs, restless legs syndrome or sleep apnea, may also develop Fibromyalgia. You may be more likely to develop Fibromyalgia if a relative also has the condition pointing to a possible genetic predisposition. Having a rheumatic disease, such as rheumatoid arthritis, lupus or ankylosing spondylitis, may cause a person to be more prone to developing Fibromyalgia.

Fibromyalgia symptoms are not restricted just to pain, but it usually has several accompanying signs and symptoms, thus making it more correctly termed **Fibromyalgia syndrome**. The other possible symptoms to this syndrome might include debilitating joint stiffness, chronic fatigue, sleep disturbance, difficulty with swallowing, bowel and bladder abnormalities, numbness and tingling in the extremities, and cognitive dysfunction. Fibromyalgia is frequently accompanied by psychiatric conditions such as depression and anxiety, and stress-related disorders such as posttraumatic stress disorder. Few people with Fibromyalgia experience all these associated symptoms, but most experience some collateral problems. Hypersensitivity affects many patients causing them discomfort in bright light, around loud noises, and intense odors.

Fibromyalgia continues to be considered a controversial diagnosis, lacking a widely accepted scientific consensus as to its cause. Not all members of the medical community regard Fibromyalgia a disease because of a frequent lack of precise abnormalities on physical examination and the absence of objective diagnostic tests or laboratory findings. *However, Fibromyalgia has been recognized as a diagnosable disorder by the American College of Rheumatology and the National Institutes of Health.*

Fibromyalgia has historically been considered to be either a musculoskeletal disease or neuropsychiatric disorder. Although there is to date no known or established cure for Fibromyalgia, some recent treatment plans have been demonstrated, by controlled clinical trials, to be effective in reducing symptoms. These programs include medications, behavioral interventions, patient education, and exercise.

Chapter 2

Symptoms of Fibromyalgia

Signs and symptoms of Fibromyalgia vary considerably from patient to patient depending on the triggering causes, which can include, stress, physical activity, trauma, or even the time of day. The common signs and symptoms include widespread pain, fatigue, and sleep disturbances, irritable bowel syndrome, headache and facial pain, and heightened sensory sensitivity. Fibromyalgia patients suffer pain in specific areas of the body when pressure is applied, in the back of the head, upper back and neck, upper chest, elbows, hips, knees, heels, and other areas on the body. The pain might persist for months at a time or be intermittent, and it is usually accompanied by stiffness.

Patients with Fibromyalgia may wake up tired and un-refreshed even though they seem to get sufficient of sleep. People with Fibromyalgia appear to miss the deep restorative stage of sleep. Nighttime muscle spasms in their legs, and restless legs syndrome also seem to be frequently associated with Fibromyalgia.

The constipation, diarrhea, abdominal pain and bloating associated with irritable bowel syndrome are commonly present in people suffering Fibromyalgia. Patients who have Fibromyalgia also frequently suffer headaches and facial pain that may be accompanied by tenderness or stiffness in their neck and shoulders.

Temporomandibular joint or TMJ dysfunction, which affects the jaw joints and surrounding muscles with severe pain, may also appear in people suffering Fibromyalgia. Furthermore, patients with Fibromyalgia may be hypersensitive to odors, noises, bright lights, and touch.

Other common signs and symptoms include depression, numbness, or tingling sensations in the hands and feet known as paresthesias. They frequently suffer difficulty concentrating and focusing, mood swings, chest pain, as well as dry eyes, skin and mouth. In addition some patients experience painful menstrual periods, vertigo and anxiety.

Given all these possible signs and symptoms associated with Fibromyalgia, the main Fibromyalgia symptoms are the usual deep muscle pain, painful tender points, morning stiffness, and sleep problems.

Review the Common Symptoms of Fibromyalgia

Common symptoms of Fibromyalgia or the Fibromyalgia Syndrome, or FMS, may include:

- ❖ Pain deep in muscles, joints and tendons
- ❖ Morning stiffness
- ❖ Sleep problems
- ❖ Swelling, numbness, and tingling in hands, arms, feet, and legs known as paresthesias.
- ❖ Tender trigger points
- ❖ Concentration and memory problems, known as "fibro fog"

❖ Depression
❖ Anxiety
❖ Chronic fatigue
❖ Headaches
❖ Irritable bowel syndrome
❖ Painful menstrual cramps
❖ Urinary symptoms

The widespread body pain is the most characteristic symptom of Fibromyalgia occurring in over 97% of patients diagnosed with the disease. It is this characteristic incessant body pain that usually brings a person to see his or her doctor.

The joint pain of Fibromyalgia differs from the joint pain of osteoarthritis in that Fibromyalgia pain is most often felt over the entire body. The pain of Fibromyalgia can be a deep, sharp, dull, throbbing, or aching and is felt in the muscles, tendons, and ligaments around the joints rather than *in the joints* like arthritis. Fibromyalgia pain may come and go and also tends to travel throughout the body, differentiating it from arthritis pain.

Painful Tender Trigger Points Accompany Fibromyalgia Pain

Accompanying the deep muscle soreness and body aches, people with Fibromyalgia have painful tender *trigger points*, which are localized areas of tenderness around joints that hurt when pressed with a finger or are subjected to pressure from objects. It is the tissue around the joints rather than the joints themselves that hurts when touched. These tender trigger points are usually superficial, located under the surface of the skin rather than deep. The locations of the tender trigger points are not random, but are often in predictable places on the body. In a person not suffering from Fibromyalgia applying pressure to points on the body, he or she would just feel pressure. For the person with Fibromyalgia, pressing the trigger points even lightly is extremely painful.

Chronic Fatigue Frequently Accompanies Fibromyalgia Syndrome

In addition to pain and trigger points, chronic fatigue is often a major complaint. Fatigue in Fibromyalgia is a lingering, ever present tiredness that is more constant and limiting than what would be expected, even being present after sufficient sleep. Patients report the fatigue of Fibromyalgia as being similar to the symptoms of flu. Fibromyalgia patients, often complain of fatigue on arising in the morning, after mild activity such as grocery shopping, cleaning, or cooking dinner, feeling too fatigued to start a project such as folding clothes or ironing, almost always too fatigued to exercise, too fatigued for sex, or too fatigued to function adequately at work.

Sleep Disturbances Are Common In Fibromyalgia

Sleep disturbances are very common among the great majority of people with Fibromyalgia. While people they may not have difficulty falling asleep, their sleep is light and easily disturbed. Many awaken in the morning feeling exhausted and un-refreshed even after eight or more hours of sleep. They turn and jerk, often complaining of bedding causing pain on their trigger points. These sleep disturbances help cause the constant state of fatigue.

Sleep studies are one area where Fibromyalgia patients show results differing from people with out the disease. During sleep studies, individuals with Fibromyalgia are constantly interrupted by bursts of brain activity similar to the activity occurring in the brain when they are awake. Sleep lab testing done on individuals with Fibromyalgia have shown that Fibromyalgia patients experience interruptions in their deep sleep periods, limiting the amount of time they spend in important deep sleep. As a result, their body is unable to rejuvenate and refresh itself.

Morning Stiffness Affect
Most Fibromyalgia Patients

More than 75% of people diagnosed with Fibromyalgia feel stiffness in the morning when they awaken and get up. The stiffness widely affects the muscles and joints of the back, arms, and legs. Patients feel the need to "loosen up" after getting out of bed before they feel they can begin their usual day's activities. In some cases the morning stiffness may last only a few minutes, but generally, it is very noticeable for more than 15 to 20 minutes each day, and in some cases the stiffness lasts for hours, sometimes it seems to be present all day.

While most people occasionally feel stiff when they first awaken, the stiffness associated with Fibromyalgia is much more than a minor aching or limitation of motion. Patients with Fibromyalgia have the same feeling of morning stiffness that people feel with many types of arthritis, especially rheumatoid or inflammatory arthritis.

Depression May Be
A Fibromyalgia Symptom

Certainly all depression is not a sign of impending Fibromyalgia, but it is a key symptom for many people with Fibromyalgia. Approximately one out of every four patients with Fibromyalgia has a concurrent major depression. Also, many people with Fibromyalgia have a long, or even a lifetime history of depression.

Stress from the constant pain and fatigue can cause anxiety as well as depression. Also, the chronic pain can result in a person being less active and thus becoming more withdrawn, often leading to depression. Furthermore, many patients with Fibromyalgia tell of having great difficulty concentrating on their work and of impaired short-term memory, which tends to depress them all the more.

Swelling Or Tingling In Hands, Feet, And Extremities In Fibromyalgia

Neurological complaints, such as paresthesias, numbness, tingling, and burning are often present in Fibromyalgia. Though the causes of these feelings is unclear, the numbness or tingling sensations in the hands, arms, or legs are felt by more than half of the Fibromyalgia patients. These sensations usually happen at irregular times, and when they do occur, they may last a few minutes or they may remain constant. These sensations can be very bothersome, but they are not often severely limiting.

Chronic Headaches May Accompany Fibromyalgia Syndrome

Chronic headaches, including recurrent migraine and/or tension-type headaches, are quite common in about 75% of people with Fibromyalgia. These often debilitating headaches can pose a serious problem in a person's ability to cope with and manage FMS. These headaches may start with a pain or stiffness in the neck and upper part of the back. They spread from a tightness and contraction of the muscles of the neck, which results in a tension-type headaches or muscle-contraction headaches. They may also be caused by tender or trigger points over the back of the head and neck. However, other medical problems can cause headaches and should be properly diagnosed and treated by a doctor. Chronic headaches require evaluation and diagnosis to find their specific cause.

Irritable Bowel Syndrome
May Be A Symptom of Fibromyalgia

Constipation, diarrhea, frequent abdominal pain, abdominal gas, continuous belching, and nausea are symptoms frequently found in between 40% to 70% of patients with Fibromyalgia. Acid reflux or gastro-esophageal reflux disease (GERD) also occurs with the same high frequency. But these symptoms may have an independent cause in patients with or without Fibromyalgia and should be thoroughly investigated and diagnosed by a gastroenterologist.

Urinary Frequency Is Often A Symptom of Fibromyalgia

Feeling a frequent urge to urinate or urinary frequency, painful urination, or incontinence may be present in about 25% or more of the cases of Fibromyalgia. Since other bladder or kidney problems may cause these symptoms, such as infection, check with your physician to be sure no other causative problems are present.

Severe Menstrual Cramps May Affect Women With Fibromyalgia

Severely painful menstrual cramps occur in 30% to 40% or more of women with Fibromyalgia. These cramps are usually recurrent for years.

Restless Legs Syndrome May Occur With Fibromyalgia

Restless legs syndrome causes discomfort in the legs, especially the areas of the legs below the knees, and the feet, and is especially bothersome at night. The feeling may be painful, but most often it is described as the need to move the legs to make them comfortable, but whatever position the discomfort remains. Restless legs syndrome interrupts sleep as the person tosses and turns, trying to find a comfortable position. As with other symptoms, restless legs syndrome can be found alone and in itself does not constitute a diagnosis of Fibromyalgia.

Chapter 3

Causes of Fibromyalgia

Doctors and researchers do not know what causes Fibromyalgia, but the current thinking centers on a *"central sensitization"* theory. This theory considers that people with Fibromyalgia have a lower threshold for pain because of the increased sensitivity in the brain to pain signals. Researchers believe repeated nerve stimulation and impulses actually cause the brains of Fibromyalgia patients to change. This change may be due to an abnormal increase in levels of certain chemicals, *the neurotransmitters,* in the brain that signal pain as excessive. In addition, the brain's pain receptors seem to overreact to pain signals. What actually initiates this process of central nervous system hyper-sensitization is not yet known or understood.

It is quite likely that a number of factors contribute to the development of *Fibromyalgia Syndrome*, or *FMS*. These causes of Fibromyalgia might be related to sleep disturbances, injury, infection, abnormalities of the autonomic or sympathetic nervous system and changes in muscle metabolism. Psychological stress and hormonal changes may also be possible causes or triggers of Fibromyalgia Syndrome.

Investigators are constantly looking at various explanations for the causes of Fibromyalgia Syndrome. While some, for example, are exploring hormonal disturbances and chemical imbalances that affect nerve signaling, others believe Fibromyalgia, because of its deep muscle pain, is linked to stress, illness, or perhaps trauma. Other researchers and practitioners think there is a hereditary cause, and some say there is no explanation or real cause. But while there is no clear consensus about what causes Fibromyalgia, most researchers believe the Fibromyalgia Syndrome results not from a single event but from a combination of many physical and emotional causes.

Additional Theories With Reference To Causes Of Fibromyalgia

Some researchers and practitioners have suggested that a lower level brain neurotransmitter called **serotonin** leads to lowered pain thresholds and an increased sensitivity to pain. The lowered pain thresholds in Fibromyalgia patients may be caused by the reduced effectiveness of the body's natural **endorphins**, the bodies own natural analgesic and the increased presence of a chemical called **substance P**, which amplifies our pain signals. There have been some worthy of note studies that link Fibromyalgia to sudden trauma to the brain and/or spinal cord. However, keep in mind, all theories regarding the causes Fibromyalgia are so far speculative.

As we have mentioned before, Fibromyalgia is far more common in women than in men. Some studies have shown that women have approximately seven times less serotonin in the brain than men on the average. That might explain why Fibromyalgia syndrome, or FMS, is far more common in women than in men.

Another theory proposes that Fibromyalgia is caused by

biochemical changes in the body, which may be related to hormonal variations or changes due to menopause. It has been noted that some people with Fibromyalgia have low levels of human growth hormone, which could contribute to the muscle pain so prevalent in the disease.

A large number of researchers and practitioners theorize and believe that stress is a strong factor in the cause of Fibromyalgia. Some scientists believe that because Fibromyalgia Syndrome is often accompanied by depression, there may be a link between the two, however, today, mental health issues are not thought to cause Fibromyalgia. More likely chronic pain, however, can cause feelings of anxiety and depression, which may worsen Fibromyalgia symptoms.

Another theory suggests that muscular trauma or severe strain might leads to an ongoing cycle of pain and fatigue. Related to this are the theories that FMS might be caused due to poor physical fitness. It might partly explain why women, who are not as strong physically as men, more often suffer from FMS.

Most people with Fibromyalgia Syndrome experience insomnia or sleep disorders. Their sleep is non-restorative sleep that is light and un-refreshing. This raises the question, "Does insomnia or sleep disorders cause Fibromyalgia?" Disordered sleep might lead to lower levels of serotonin, which results in increased pain sensitivity, and interestingly researchers have created a lower pain threshold in women by depriving them of sleep, somewhat simulating Fibromyalgia. However most practitioners suspect that FMS causes sleep disorders rather that the reverse. This remains an interesting area of study and research.

Is Fibromyalgia Hereditary?

Like other rheumatic and autoimmune diseases, Fibromyalgia seemingly could be the result of a genetic tendency passed from mothers to off springs. According to the belief of some researchers a person's genes may determine the way his or her body processes painful stimuli. People with Fibromyalgia may have a gene or genes that cause them to react intensely to stimuli that most other people would not perceive as painful or too intense. If they do indeed exist, these genes have not been isolated or identified as yet.

There is a high aggregation of Fibromyalgia in families. The mode of inheritance is currently unknown, but research has demonstrated that Fibromyalgia is potentially associated with genes in the serotoninergic, dopaminergic, and catecholaminergic systems. More about these chemical differences will be explained below. However, these genetics are not specific for Fibromyalgia and are associated with a variety of allied disorders, such as chronic fatigue syndrome, irritable bowel syndrome, and with chronic chemical depression.

It is theorized that when a person with this genetic tendency is exposed to triggering emotional or physical stressors, such as a traumatic crisis, severe injury, or a serious illness, there is a change in the body's response to such stresses, which can result in a greater sensitivity of the entire body to pain.

Dopamine dysfunction

The "dopamine dysfunction theory of Fibromyalgia causation suggests that the chief abnormality responsible for symptoms associated with FMS is a disorder of the normal dopamine neurotransmission. This Insufficiency of dopamine is called **hypodopaminergia**. Dopamine is a pain perception and natural analgesia transmitter. Furthermore there is also strong evidence for a role of dopamine in restless leg syndrome, which is a condition found frequently in patients with Fibromyalgia. Some Fibromyalgia patients positively responded in controlled scientific studies to pramipexole, a dopamine agonist that selectively stimulates dopamine D2/D3 receptors and is used to treat both Parkinson's disease and restless leg syndrome.

Abnormal Serotonin Metabolism

As early as 1975, researchers hypothesized that serotonin, a neurotransmitter that regulates sleep patterns, mood, concentration, and pain, might be involved in the cause of Fibromyalgia-associated symptoms. In 1992, decreased serotonin metabolites in patient blood samples, and their cerebrospinal fluid was reported. However, selective serotonin reuptake inhibitors have met with limited success in alleviating the symptoms of the disorder. In controlled trials funded by Eli Lily, Duloxetine (Cymbalta), originally used to treat depression and painful diabetic neuropathy, was demonstrated to relieve Fibromyalgia symptoms in some women, however male subjects failed significant improvement. Nonetheless, the Food and Drug Administration regulators approved the drug for the treatment of Fibromyalgia in June 2008. The relevance of serotonin metabolism remains a matter of debate.

Deficient Growth Hormone Secretion

Levels of hormones under the direct or indirect control of growth hormone including IGF-1, cortisol, and neuropeptide Y may be abnormal in people with FMS but supplementing growth hormone in patients has not proven to have great effects. There is disagreement about the role of growth hormone in Fibromyalgia, and requires much more study.

Stress

Stress may be an important precipitating factor in the development of Fibromyalgia. Fibromyalgia is frequently accompanied with stress-related disorders such as chronic fatigue, posttraumatic stress disorder, irritable bowel syndrome, and depression. Other researchers and practitioners have suggested that, because exposure to stressful conditions might a triggering mechanism to the development of the Fibromyalgia Syndrome.

Psychological factors

There is strong and compelling evidence that major depression is associated with fibromyalgia. A comprehensive review into the relationship between FMS and major depressive disorders found substantial similarities in neuroendocrine abnormalities, psychological characteristics, physical symptoms, and treatments between fibromyalgia and major chemical depressions.

Physical trauma

There has been demonstration that severe trauma

and some surgery can trigger the onset of FMS. Neck trauma especially, seems to increase the risk of developing Fibromyalgia. In these cases the patient is often labeled as having Traumatic Fibromyalgia Syndrome.

Apparent Risk Factors For Fibromyalgia

Risk factors for a specific disease are distinct characteristics researchers have identified that may increase a potential patient's chance of getting that illness or precipitating the disease. The common risk factors risk researchers have identified for Fibromyalgia include:

❖ gender usually female

❖ genetic disposition may be inherited

❖ menopause, loss of estrogen, or other hormonal changes

❖ poor physical conditioning generally

❖ surgery, or chronic or serious illness

❖ trauma to the brain or spinal cord after an injury, accident, illness

❖ emotional stress

❖ depression

❖ anxiety

Also some women have Fibromyalgia with certain diseases, such as   osteoarthritis, rheumatoid arthritis, systemic lupus Erythematosis (SLE), or other autoimmune diseases.

It needs to be noted that there are many people with Fibromyalgia Syndrome who have none of these traits, or without any notable underlying disease.

In summary

There is no single theory that explains the cause of Fibromyalgia, nor is it understood what causes Fibromyalgia to flare up. Whatever causes the unending pain, tender points, and insomnia or sleep problems, they are certain to increase the fatigue and depression you feel. This, in turn, can lead to increased anxiety, reduced activity, and greater pain. It becomes a vicious cycle. Disordered sleep, and the lack of REM sleep, can reduce your energy levels. Over time, it can lead to a decrease in the body's ability to repair damaged tissues. The lowered activity level caused by lack of sleep and pain in turn decreases physical fitness and reduces limberness. More pain and inactivity follows.

Fortunately, once your doctor makes a proper Fibromyalgia diagnosis, effective treatment for Fibromyalgia can be started. At present there is no known cure for Fibromyalgia, but you can manage the symptoms and preserve your quality of life.

Again, **Fibromyalgia is not a life threatening disease**.

Chapter 4

Diagnosis of Fibromyalgia

Fibromyalgia is a difficult diagnosis to make because there isn't a specific diagnostic laboratory test. The fact is that it is most often a diagnosis by process of elimination. Before making a diagnosis of Fibromyalgia doctors usually, go through numerous medical tests, including blood tests and X-rays, only to have the results come back normal. These tests usually help to rule out other conditions, such as rheumatoid arthritis, lupus, and multiple sclerosis, but they cannot confirm Fibromyalgia.

Finally, the **American College of Rheumatology** has established general guidelines for Fibromyalgia study and diagnosis. Following these guidelines, to be diagnosed with Fibromyalgia the patient must have experienced widespread aching and pain for at minimum three months, and have at least eleven locations on the body that are abnormally tender under relatively mild, firm pressure. Of particular interest are specific points of tenderness on the patient's head and upper body. However not all doctors agree with these guidelines feeling that these criteria are far too rigid.

Fibromyalgia Diagnosis and Misdiagnosis

There is no single test that altogether shows if someone has Fibromyalgia; the fact is there is still debate over what should be considered essential diagnostic criteria, and whether objective diagnosis is possible. The difficulty with diagnosing Fibromyalgia is that, in most cases, laboratory testing appears normal and that many of the symptoms mimic those of other autoimmune conditions such as arthritis, gout, lupus, or numerous other diseases with similar symptoms. In general, most doctors diagnose patients with a process called **differential diagnosis**, meaning that doctors consider all of the possible things that might be wrong with the patient based on the patient's symptoms, gender, age, geographic location, medical history and other factors, then narrow down the diagnosis to the most likely one by process of elimination. The most widely accepted set of classification, which are known informally as "the ACR 1990", define Fibromyalgia according to the presence of the following criteria:

A history of widespread pain lasting more than three months—affecting all four quadrants of the body meaning both sides, and above and below the waist.

Tender points must number at least 11 or more of these trigger points for Fibromyalgia to be considered.

It should be noted that the ACR criteria for classification of patients were originally established as inclusion criteria for research purposes and were not intended for clinical diagnosis, but have now become the *de facto* diagnostic criteria in the clinical setting. Also, it must be noted that the number of tender points that may be active at any one time may vary with time and circumstance.

A doctor needs to make an accurate diagnosis of Fibromyalgia. Unfortunately, Fibromyalgia is regularly misunderstood. Despite all the latest information about FMS with its severe muscle pain, unrelenting fatigue and sleep problems, and feelings of anxiety and depression, doctors are still misdiagnosing this common pain disorder. Because Fibromyalgia is so multifaceted some patients are getting a diagnosis for the wrong conditions such as chronic fatigue syndrome, arthritis, or some other pain-involving problem.

There are no clinical or scientific measures, such as laboratory tests, X-rays, or devices that can prove you have Fibromyalgia. In the past, millions of Fibromyalgia patients were misdiagnosed as having depression, inflammatory arthritis such as rheumatoid or lupus, chronic myofascial pain, or chronic fatigue syndrome, among other diseases with similar symptoms. Though there are many similarities between Fibromyalgia and chronic fatigue syndrome and between Fibromyalgia and arthritis and other autoimmune diseases, Fibromyalgia is different; it is a distinct condition that needs an accurate diagnosis and unique and appropriate treatment.

Most laboratory tests are not very useful by themselves for diagnosing Fibromyalgia, however they are used to rule out other possible diseases with similar symptoms. Your doctor will probably come to a diagnosis after doing a physical exam and discussing your symptoms with you. Tests may be ordered to rule out other illnesses. In other words your doctor will use a few lab tests to make sure you don't have some other, perhaps, serious medical condition.

Among the blood tests that your doctor may order is a

complete blood count, or better known as a CBC. This test measures the hemoglobin, red cells, white cells, and platelets. A complete blood count gives important information about the kinds and numbers of cells in the blood, especially red blood cells, white blood cells, and platelets. The CBC helps your doctor check for the cause of many symptoms, such as weakness, fatigue, or bruising, you may have. The CBC also helps your physician diagnose conditions, such as anemia, infection, as well as many other possible disorders.

Your physician may also ask for other tests, including kidney and liver studies, and blood chemistries. Your doctor will probably want to know your cholesterol level and other fats in your blood, calcium levels, and more. In addition, your doctor may run thyroid tests to see if your thyroid is overactive or underactive. A red blood cell sedimentation rate may be ordered as an index of possible inflammation in the body. In rheumatoid and other forms of arthritis, this test is abnormal; it may also be abnormal with some infections, but interestingly in cases of osteoarthritis and Fibromyalgia, it is usually normal.

Another test your physician might order is a rheumatoid factor. This blood test measures for an abnormal protein in the blood and is positive for 70% to 80% percent of patients with rheumatoid arthritis. However, this blood test can also be positive in healthy individuals and is negative in 20% to 30% of people suffering with rheumatoid arthritis. Also, your doctor may test for anti-nuclear antibody, or ANA. Like rheumatoid factor, ANA is an abnormal antibody in the blood commonly found with **systemic lupus**. Systemic lupus is more common in women, especially younger women, and can cause pain and fatigue similar to Fibromyalgia, but unlike FMS systemic lupus may also cause internal organ problems, such as kidney disease, heart disease, or problems in the brain.

X-rays may be ordered to rule out other diseases because in the case of Fibromyalgia, X-rays of painful areas will not show abnormality. If you have another problem, such as arthritis, then there would likely be some abnormalities on the X-rays to indicate what type of arthritis you have. In other words, any X-ray changes are *not* due to Fibromyalgia.

Ask questions of your physician. Speak openly with him or her in order to fully understand the overall results of the diagnostic process. Have your physician explain completely the findings from the physical exam and laboratory testing, and any X-rays that might have been taken. Thorough communications will help you understand your Fibromyalgia. Ask any questions you may have about FMS, its symptoms, and all your treatment options.

Summary Of The Diagnostic Guidelines for Fibromyalgia

After ruling out other possible medical problems, through physical exam and laboratory tests, and perhaps X-ray studies, your physician will consider whether your condition meets two defining Fibromyalgia criteria:

Has there been widespread pain in all four quadrants of your body, upper and lower, left and right, for a minimum of three months?

Do you have tenderness or pain in at least 11 of 18 specific tender points when pressure is applied?

To be thorough in making the correct diagnosis of Fibromyalgia, your physician will probably do the following six things:

❖ check for widespread pain

❖ evaluate trigger points

❖ ask about fatigue

❖ inquire about sleep disturbances

❖ evaluate your level of stress

❖ test for depression

If you are indeed diagnosed as having Fibromyalgia, your physician will discuss a specific and multifaceted treatment program with you. That program may include medications, exercise, stress reduction, sleep strategies, and more. Staying on this program will help ease your Fibromyalgia symptoms so you can more easily cope, and reclaim an active life doing the things you want to do.

Chapter 5

Treatments Of Fibromyalgia

The main emphasis in treating Fibromyalgia is toward minimizing symptoms and improving general health and function. This care generally includes medication and self-care. Since the Fibromyalgia Syndrome encompasses a variety of symptoms, not necessarily suffered by all patients, treatment for this disease requires a specific treatment plan for virtually every patient. One plan does not fit all.

For Fibromyalgia, as with numerous other medically unexplained syndromes, there is no known cure or universally accepted treatment, and FMS treatment is typically aimed at symptom management. Improved understanding of the pathophysiology of Fibromyalgia has led to improvements in treatment, which may include prescription medication, behavioral intervention, exercise, and alternative and supplementary medication. Indeed, integrated treatment plans that incorporate medication, patient education, aerobic exercise and cognitive-behavioral therapy have been shown to be effective in alleviating pain and the many other FMS symptoms.

Your physician may prescribe pain medication and/or antidepressants to help reduce or end the pain, fatigue, depression, and anxiety that comes with this disease. In addition, your doctor may recommend physical therapy, moist heat, regular aerobic exercise, relaxation, and stress reduction to help you self-manage your FMS symptoms. There is no one magic pill that treats or cures Fibromyalgia. A multidisciplinary approach that uses both medication and alternative or lifestyle strategies is needed and seems to work best to treat the many Fibromyalgia Syndrome symptoms. Along with deep muscle pain and painful tender points of FMS, fatigue is a key symptom of Fibromyalgia and can be severely debilitating. Not only do FMS patients often feel totally exhausted and weak, but also bed rest does not seem to help. Many people with Fibromyalgia report sleeping up to eight or ten hours at night yet they feel like they haven't slept at all.

Fibromyalgia fatigue is often described as crippling, exhausting, and flu-like. You may experience fatigue on arising, even after ten hours of bed rest. Many people with FMS have disturbances in their deep level or most restful sleep time. The fatigue with FMS often coincides with mood disturbances, anxiety, or depression. People with Fibromyalgia may describe their sleep as un-refreshing or light. Some people with Fibromyalgia complain of pain and achiness around the joints in the neck, shoulder, back, and hips making it even more difficult to sleep, thus worsening their feelings of constant sleepiness and fatigue.

There are similarities between Fibromyalgia fatigue and chronic fatigue syndrome, which is a condition primarily characterized by ongoing, debilitating fatigue. People with FMS frequently describe the fatigue they feel as "brain fatigue." a condition called "fibro fog."

There are some drugs that may help ease the chronic fatigue associated with FMS, and aerobic exercise can help ease fatigue, minimize your pain, quite often improve your quality of sleep, and improve your mood.

Exercise And Fibromyalgia

Numerous studies have shown that exercise is one of the most important treatments for Fibromyalgia. Many people with FMS are physically unfit, avoiding exercise because they fear increased pain, however, aerobic exercise and physical conditioning actually help relieve pain and depression. Regular exercise increases the body's production of endorphins, the natural painkillers that also boost mood. Starting slowly and gradually increasing the duration and intensity of exercise will help you enjoy the benefits of exercise without feeling more pain. Also, physical therapy can help relieve Fibromyalgia pain and stiffness. A licensed physical therapist can increase confidence with exercise, help relax tense muscles, and teach you more about your body and its movements.

A competent physical therapist will show you the proper way to stretch painful muscles to get optimal pain and stiffness relief. Using hydrotherapy and moist heat or ice packs along with physical therapy may ease your pain even more. Physical therapy can help you to regain control of your illness and confidence. You'll be able to focus on lifestyle changes rather than on the chronic dysfunction brought on by your disease. Regaining proper posture, which your physical therapist will also help you with, will allow more efficient muscle function. This will reduce undue fatigue and pain.

Medications And Fibromyalgia

Antidepressants are recommended as first-line drugs to treat FMS according to guidelines from the ***American***

Pain Society. These medications can affect multiple symptoms including pain, fatigue, depressed mood, and sleep disturbances. The older tricyclic and newer antidepressants usually provide effective symptom relief, but they won't totally eliminate all the pain.

More recently, Lyrica, an anti-convulsant drug, has been approved by the FDA for Fibromyalgia treatment. Lyrica reduces pain and improves daily function for some FMS patients; however, the drug's most common side effects include sleepiness and mild to moderate dizziness. Lyrica can also cause swelling and weight gain, and Lyrica may impair the ability to drive. Other anticonvulsants have also been used to treat Fibromyalgia.

Cymbalta is another drug recently approved, by the FDA for the treatment of Fibromyalgia. An antidepressant, Cymbalta belongs to a class of drugs called serotonin and norepinephrine reuptake inhibitors (SNRIs). Cymbalta's most common side effects include nausea, dry mouth, and constipation, and in some cases it can also cause insomnia and dizziness.

The FDA has also approved Savella for treating Fibromyalgia. Savella, like Cymbalta, is in the class of drugs known as SNRIs, but while it acts in the body the same way certain antidepressants do, Savella is not used to treat depression. Savella, when used to treat Fibromyalgia, has been shown to reduce pain, improve physical function, and bring about overall FMS improvement for many patients. The most common side effects of Savella are nausea, headache, constipation, dizziness, and insomnia.

Medications, which help increase restful sleep, might help treat FMS symptoms. These drugs include low doses of antidepressant medications such as amitriptyline taken before bedtime. Other classes of sleeping pills are, however, not very helpful for people who have Fibromyalgia.

Anti-inflammatory drugs, such as ibuprofen and naproxen, are not usually helpful since there is little or no inflammation with Fibromyalgia. However, they may help boost pain relief from other FMS medications. Keep in mind that anti-inflammatory drugs have many side effects, such as stomach upset, and bleeding, and in some cases may increase blood pressure. The pain reliever acetaminophen may be helpful, and it is easier on the stomach and less likely to cause drug interactions than anti-inflammatory drugs. However, acetaminophen should only be taken as recommended. Too much acetaminophen can lead to sever liver problems.

Some muscle relaxants, such as Flexeril, have been known to provide some relief of muscle pain, especially when taken at bedtime.

Steroids used to treat inflammation associated with other rheumatic conditions have been tested in people with FMS, and like other anti-inflammatory drugs, did not appear to improve symptoms. However, a steroid injection directly into a muscle spasm or trigger point may sometimes help when other treatments have failed. The number of steroid injections that can be used in a given period of time is limited.

Non-narcotic analgesics such as Ultram, are considerably stronger analgesics than acetaminophen and are commonly used to treat FMS. This narcotic-like medication acts centrally in the brain to change the sensation of pain. There is no anti-inflammatory effect, and is not as addictive as narcotics.

Many doctors prescribe benzodiazepines such as Ativan, Klonopin, Valium, Xanax, which can help to relax painful muscles, improve sleep, and relieve symptoms of restless legs syndrome. These medications tend to depress the central nervous system, resulting in sedation, skeletal muscle relaxation, and anticonvulsant activity. They can sometimes cause coma in too large doses. Benzodiazepines are addictive and must be used with caution on a short-term basis. Caution must be taken while driving or use of dangerous tools.

Powerful opioid pain medications, such as OxyContin, should only be considered if all other drugs and alternative therapies have been exhausted and there is no relief. The danger with the use of opioids is that their long-term use, as may be needed in the treatment of FMS, could lead to serious drug addiction.

Any use of medication in the treatment of FMS should be under the direction of a physician.

In addition to medication, other therapies, such as cognitive-behavioral therapy, can help develop confidence, a sense of control over your disease, and provide necessary and valuable education about your condition. Talk therapy can help you learn new self-management strategies and significantly boost your coping skills. Seeking psychological counseling may be a wise choice in your multifaceted treatment program for FMS.

Chapter 6

Alternative Treatments Can Help Fibromyalgia

You may wonder about the effectiveness of alternative therapies to ease the discomfort of Fibromyalgia pain. Many patients suffering with the chronic pain of FMS do indeed find good quality relief with alternative therapies, including the following:

Acupuncture, which some studies show may alter brain chemistry and help increase pain tolerance.

Chiropractic, which may improve pain levels, ease low back pain, and increase spinal ranges of motion.

Deep tissue massage, which appears to stimulate circulation and release chronic muscular tension.

Neuromuscular massage, which combines the basic principles of ancient Oriental therapies, such as acupressure, shiatsu, and specific hands-on deep tissue therapy to help reduce deep chronic muscle pain.

Biofeedback, which helps people learn to control the stress response and relieves chronic pain.

Meditation, which seems to produces brain waves consistent with serenity and happiness, which help to relieve anxiety, depression, and stress.

Herbal remedies, which seem to help some patients, although there are few studies on herbal remedies and FMS. Patients report improved sleep or more energy with herbal supplements such as echinacea, black cohosh, lavender, milk thistle, B vitamins, and numerous other non-prescription remedies.

Natural dietary supplements, while there are limited studies on natural dietary supplements and their benefit in treating Fibromyalgia, some patients have found relief with over-the-counter natural dietary supplements such as 5-HTP, melatonin, St. John's Wort, L-carnitine, SAM-e, and probiotics.

Patients with FMS often use medical marijuana, which can be prescribed by physicians in some states, and seems to help relieve their chronic pain and fatigue. Medical marijuana certainly doesn't cure diseases like Fibromyalgia, however, some pain experts believe it works to ease pain, help patients sleep better, and markedly improves their mood.

Managing the many and varied symptoms FMS is not easy, so it is no wonder that many patients turn to alternative therapies for relief of pain, sleep, other Fibromyalgia Syndrome and problems. Because so many patients, not just those with FMS, are using alternative therapies for all kinds of symptoms, the United States Congress has formed the **National Center for Complementary and Alternative Medicine (NCCAM)** as part of the **National Institutes of Health (NIH),** to helps evaluate alternative treatments, including supplements, and to define their effectiveness. This organization is now creating safe guidelines to help people choose appropriate alternative therapies that may help their symptoms without causing injury or illness.

How Safe And Effective Are Herbs and Supplements For FMA?

Some studies indicate that a number of medicinal herbs and natural supplements appear to help treat symptoms of Fibromyalgia. They are by no means a cure, but some do seem to relieve various FMS symptoms. Patients report that they feel better using some herbs and supplements and have recurrence of symptoms when they stop using them. To take a natural herbal and supplemental approach to FMA treatment, it's important to learn as much as you can about the therapies you consider using. Always when using herbs and supplements check with your physician to make sure they are not libel to interfere with other medications you are taking. *Some herbs, supplements, and over-the-counter products can have dangerous interactions with prescription drugs.*

5-HTP (**5-Hydroxytryptophan)** is a fundamental building block of serotonin. Serotonin is a controlling brain chemical, and serotonin levels brain play a significant role in Fibromyalgia pain. Serotonin levels are also linked with depression and sleep. Thus, 5-HTP may help both to increase deep sleep and reduce pain, as well as improve mood. However, there are some contradictory studies that show no benefit with 5-HTP.

5-HTP is usually well tolerated. It should be noted that in the late 1980s, the supplement was associated with a serious condition called eosinophilia-myalgia syndrome. It's thought, however, that a contaminant in 5-HTP led to the condition, which causes flu-like symptoms, severe muscle pain, and burning rashes, rather than the 5-HTP itself.

Melatonin is a natural hormone available as an over-the-counter supplement. It is often used to induce drowsiness and improve sleep patterns. Travelers frequently use it to combat Jet Lag. Some studies show that melatonin may be effective in treating Fibromyalgia pain. Most patients with FMS have sleep problems and fatigue, and melatonin may help relieve those symptoms. Melatonin is generally regarded as safe, having few to no side effects; however, due to the risk of daytime sleepiness, anyone taking melatonin should use caution when driving or using dangerous equipment until they know how this product affects them.

St. John's Wort is doubtfully helpful in treating Fibromyalgia. This herb is, however, often used in treating depression, and depression is commonly associated with Fibromyalgia. Several studies have shown St. John's Wort is more effective than placebo and as effective as older antidepressants called tricyclics in the treatment of mild or moderate depression. Other studies show it is as effective as selective SSRI antidepressants such as Prozac or Zoloft in treating depression. St John's Wort is more often than not well tolerated; its most common side effects are stomach upset, skin reactions, and fatigue. **An important caution**, St. John's Wort should not be mixed with antidepressants and can cause interactions with many other types of drugs. Check with your physician before taking St. John's Wort or for that matter, any supplement.

SAM-e, it's not known exactly how this supplement works in the body. Some researchers feel this natural supplement increases the levels of serotonin and dopamine, two important brain neurotransmitters. Some researchers and patients believe that SAM-e may alter mood and increase restful sleep, however, current studies do not appear to show any benefit of SAM-e over placebos in reducing the number of tender points or in alleviating depression of FMS.

L-carnitine studies are limited, but it's thought that it may give some pain relief and treat other symptoms in people with FMS. In one study, of 102 patients with Fibromyalgia researchers evaluated the effectiveness of L-carnitine, which showed significantly greater symptom improvements in the group that took L-carnitine than in the group that took a placebo. The researchers concluded, L-carnitine may provide pain relief and improvement in the general and mental health of patients with FMS, and that more studies are warranted.

Probiotics are dietary supplements, which contain potentially beneficial bacteria and/or yeasts. They may assist with the breakdown and proper absorption of food thus helping to improve digestive problems such as irritable bowel syndrome, a common symptom of Fibromyalgia. Some of the ways probiotics are used include treating diarrhea, preventing and treating infections of the urinary tract or female genitals, and treating irritable bowel syndrome. There are few side effects of taking probiotics and they are usually mild and limited to gas or bloating.

Among other herbs and natural supplements that people say have helped FMS symptoms are Echinacea, black cohosh, cayenne, lavender, milk thistle, and B vitamins. There are no definitive studies on the efficacy of these natural therapies. **Before taking any herb or supplement for Fibromyalgi; talk to your physician and/or your pharmacist about possible side effects, or herb-drug interactions.** Furthermore, **herbal therapies are not recommended for pregnant women, children, the elderly, or those patients who may have weakened immune systems.** In addition, realize that some herbs have sedative or blood-thinning qualities, which may dangerously interact with anti-inflammatory painkillers or other pain medications, or blood thinning prescription drugs.

Chapter 7

Fibromyalgia and Exercise

If you have FMS with its painful tender trigger points, deep muscle pain, and chronic fatigue, starting a program of exercise is probably the last thing on your mind. Yet exercise, whether it is daily walks, stretching, swimming, yoga, tai chi, or Pilates, low-impact exercise programs can keep you get fit in spite of your Fibromyalgia, and to your surprise, it may help reduce pain as well.

Exercise is essential for keeping muscles strong and flexible, controlling your weight, improving your sleep and mood, and helping you stay active in all facets of life. Exercise and other activities allow FMS patients to have more control over Fibromyalgia and the amount of pain and other symptoms they feel. For most patients, range of motion, strengthening, and aerobic conditioning exercises are safe and necessary.

Exercise helps restore the body's neurochemical balance and initiates a positive emotional state of mind. Regular exercise slows down the heart-racing adrenaline associated with stress, and it also boosts levels of natural endorphins, the body's natural pain-fighting chemical. Endorphins also help to reduce anxiety, stress, and depression.

Exercise tends to boosts serotonin levels in people with Fibromyalgia. Serotonin, as you will recall, is a neurotransmitter in the brain that scientists have found often to be reduced in Fibromyalgia patients. Neurotransmitters in the brain are the chemicals that send specific messages from one brain cell to another. While only a small percentage of all serotonin is located in the brain, this neurotransmitter seems to play a fundamental role in mediating moods. Studies have found that too much stress can lead to permanently low levels of serotonin, which in turn, can create aggression, anxiety, depression, and mood swings. Increased level of serotonin in the brain is associated with a calming, anxiety-reducing effect. In some cases it's also associated with drowsiness, which helps alleviate sleep problems. Stabilizing serotonin level in the brain is associated with a positive mood state and feeling good. The lack of adequate exercise and generalized inactivity can make worse your low serotonin levels.

Women, it appears, may have a greater sensitivity to changes in this brain chemical. Their mood swings during the menstrual cycle, menopause, or following the birth of a child may be hormonally induced through the action of their hormones on neurotransmitters. Also, various other factors such as sunlight, certain carbohydrate foods, and exercise can have a positive effect on serotonin. Exercise appears to act as a natural tranquilizer by helping to boost serotonin in the brain.

Studies have shown that exercise triggers the release of epinephrine and norepinephrine, two hormones that are known to boost alertness. For those who feel frequently stressed, exercise will help to desensitize the body to many of the ill effects of stress.

Other Benefits Of Exercise
For Patients With Fibromyalgia

Regular exercise benefits people with FMS by the following:

- ❖ burning calories helps making your weight control easier
- ❖ improves your range-of-motion to painful muscles and joints
- ❖ improves your self-esteem and outlook on life
- ❖ improves your quality of sleep
- ❖ improves your sense of well-being
- ❖ increases your aerobic capacity
- ❖ improves your cardiovascular health
- ❖ increases your energy
- ❖ places some control of healing in your hands
- ❖ reduces your anxiety levels and depression
- ❖ relieves your stress associated with a chronic disease
- ❖ stimulates your growth hormone secretion
- ❖ stimulates the secretion of endorphins in your body
- ❖ strengthens your bones
- ❖ strengthens your muscles
- ❖ relieves much of your pain

Types of Exercises That Work Best for Fibromyalgia Symptoms

Exercises such as walking, swimming and water aerobics, strength training, and stretching activities are very effective at improving physical, emotional, and social function for FMS patients. They also are an effective adjunct relieving symptoms and in women with Fibromyalgia who are also being treated with medication. Aquatic exercise programs, such as water aerobics and swimming are effective in reducing symptoms and improving the health-related quality of life of the participants, especially for those patients who have difficulty walking. Your exercise program, should especially focus on three major types of exercise:

Range-of-motion and stretching exercises. These types of exercises involve your moving your joints as far as they will go through its full range of motion, but without causing you pain. Range-of-motion exercises and/or stretching will help you maintain flexibility in your muscle groups. Again, stretching should not be pushed past a point of discomfort. Talk to your physician or physical therapist about range-of-motion exercises. They can explain how to do these exercises properly, giving you some guidance if you have difficulty performing proper stretching.

Endurance or conditioning exercises. When you increase your endurance capacity with cardiovascular types of exercise, such as walking, biking, or swimming, you do more than simply strengthen your muscles. You also condition your body, tone your muscles, build coordination, efficiency of motion, and endurance. These endurance exercises help with weight control, and build self-esteem. When you start your exercise program seek guidance from your physician and a competent trainer.

Strengthening exercises. Strengthening workouts and exercises help to build strong muscles and tendons needed to support your joints. Some patients report that strengthening exercises improve other FMS symptoms. Again, be cautious and seek guidance from a competent trainer so as not to hurt yourself when doing your strengthening exercises. A personal trainer or fitness expert can explain how to use resistance machines and free weights, starting slowly and increasing as you build your strength. Improving your general strength and fitness is perhaps the most important part of your multifaceted treatment program.

Low-impact aerobic exercises tend to improve symptoms and restore muscle strength in people with Fibromyalgia.

These type helpful exercises include:

Yoga, is an ancient form of exercise that can reduce stress and relieve muscular tension or pain by improving both range of motion and strength. When you are on the job or at home practicing yoga for FMS when you are feeling tense or anxious may help you reduce stress and avoid the risk of injury

Tai chi is an ancient Asian form of exercise useful for FMS patients. Tai chi uses a series of flowing, graceful movements that can give you a good workout and stretching regimen as well as improving your balance. Tai chi participants increase their sense of balance, reducing their fear of falling. They can bend and move easier, and are better able to do their household tasks and chores. Tai chi can keep your back flexible and strong thus improving your ability to cope with your FMS.

Pilates is a newer form of exercise, which focuses on your breathing and strengthening of your torso muscles. With Pilates, a specially trained instructor will help you work on the postural muscles that are essential to supporting your spine.

Water Therapy Helps People With Fibromyalgia If you have FMS, water therapy can give you good results especially if you have difficulty walking. But even patients who have no problem walking or doing other exercises, swimming, and water therapy is an ideal workout. Water therapy will strengthen and condition you as you move your body against the water's resistance. Water supports your weight during movement, which makes it low impact and helps alleviate any excess stress on muscles and joints. Water alleviates the forces of gravity and provides buoyancy as well as mild resistance providing a gentle form of conditioning.

There are usually water aerobic classes offered at most

pools and health facilities with pools. Joining such a class will not only provide you with a great exercise program, but also will find you new friends.

Walking Is A Great Exercise For FMS Patients

If you've been a sedentary person the idea of starting an exercise program may be intimidating to you. You see all those folks out there jogging, running marathons, biking, playing tennis, racquetball and participating in triathlons ... well you say you want no part of all that pain and effort. Well, we've got good news for you. The **"no pain, no gain" bit is a myth.** A great exercise program can be based strictly on walking. That's not to say you shouldn't participate in other exercise activities. On the contrary we advocate you participate in as many exercise or athletic activities as you desire. Cross training in several forms of exercise is especially good for FMS patients as it provides variety, reducing the tedium of the same workout day after day.

Regardless of whatever other activities you participate in, none can replace your walking program for its absolute perfect benefit to you physically, mentally, and aerobically! The fact is that walking is humankind's most perfect aerobic exercise and by itself could be all the exercise you need to become and stay physically fit and in control of your FMS for the rest of your life. Other exercise activities can benefit you in other ways but none can replace a good walking program for total conditioning; not biking, swimming, running, jogging, tennis, racquet ball, aerobic dance or calisthenics. Now if you really can't exercise walk due to some debilitating physical reason, then the above mentioned exercises will benefit you and help you control your Fibromyalgia.

A walking program has the additional advantage of being accessible to almost everyone anywhere. It requires no special equipment, club membership, expensive investment, special clothing other than comfortable shoes, and special athletic skills are not a necessary.

For those of you who might be skeptical of the benefits of walking as your sole (no pun intended) exercise program, consider the following:

1. Walking is humankind's most natural exercise at any age. Of all exercises it is the safest and least traumatic to body and joints. We've been designed to walk great distances at remarkable speeds. Running was meant only for short spurts during the hunt or emergencies. We weren't designed or built to withstand the punishment of long continuous running or jogging which require lifting the body weight completely off the ground and landing on bent knees with each jarring stride.

2. Walking exercises the entire body and mind. It utilizes the upper body more than running and the legs far more than swimming. In a vigorous, brisk walk there is virtually no muscle group in your body at rest. And walking stimulates mental and creative activity as well as reducing stress.

3. Walking will develop your endurance within safe boundaries faster than any other aerobic sport. No other sport can provide you with the benefits you will

be getting from your walking program in as short a time as a week from now.

4. Your waking program will give you the best cardiovascular/cardiopulmonary (aerobic) workout you can get and with the greatest margin of safety.

5. Walking can be done by virtually anyone, anytime, anywhere. It is probably the most indulged in sport in the world. Over 40% of Americans will tell you that walking is their main source of exercise ... and Americans are newcomers to the sport.

6. Walking is a family sport, one of the few that all ages can participate in equally and together.

7. We call walking a sport because it is a competitive event even to the Olympic level should, you want to pursue it. Race walking is becoming popular throughout the United States as it has been in other parts of the world for decades. Competition is usually broken down into age groups so competition can be pursued at all ages into the eighties and older. Races are also divided into men's and women's divisions and are usually broken down into 5, 10, 30 and 50 kilometer events. It is interesting to note that an Olympic or World Class race walker is among the best conditioned athletes in the world.

8. If you're not interested in that kind of competition ... and most of us aren't ... the competition you'll have against yourself will be all you need to keep you going toward ever increasing goals.

9. You'll probably burn more calories, exercise your heart, lungs and circulation better, lose more weight and develop your body and mind further than you could in any other activity. In addition walking will lower your blood pressure, reduce stress and cholesterol levels and take off up to one pound of fat a week even if you don't alter your eating habits.

Sound too good to be true?
You've heard nothing yet!

1. It reduces the likelihood of cardiovascular and cerebrovascular disease by increasing the blood flow and size and tone of the vessels.

2. It strengthens the muscles of the body including the heart muscle and makes them work more efficiently.

3. It slows the heart rate by increasing the stroke volume, the volume of blood the heart is able to pump with one contraction.

4. It tends to reduce the height to which arterial pressure rises during exercise and stress.

5. It encourages collateral circulation to the heart muscle. This can dramatically increase your chances of surviving a coronary occlusion were it to happen.

6. It reduces depositing of storage fat.

7. It improves digestion and elimination of body wastes.

8. It increases the oxygen supply to the brain and increases mental sharpness. It potentiates creative thought processes.

9. It tends to retard the aging process and gives a more youthful appearance.

10. It aids lymphatic circulation and blood circulation in general.

11. It stimulates the metabolism and the effect continues burning calories for hours after the cessation of exercise.

12. It increases respiratory capacity and aerobic power.

13. It benefits body growth and recovery from trauma.

14. It reduces blood fat or triglyceride levels.

15. It reduces insomnia and provides for better relaxation.

16. It reduces the incidence of minor illnesses, allergies, headaches and abdominal problems.

17. It improves coordination by activating neurotransmitters and training muscle fibers.

18. It increases flexibility of the joints and muscles and thus reduces aches and pains in the back, neck, and other body joints.

19. It circulates more oxygen to all body tissues.

20. It creates a better balance between oxygen required by the tissues and the oxygen made more readily available through exercise.

21. It tones up the glandular systems and increases thyroid gland output.

22. It increases the production of red blood cells by the bone marrow.

23. It increases the ability to store and utilize nutrients which increases endurance.

24. It augments the alkaline reserve of the body which can be significant in an emergency requiring extended effort.

25. It gives a feeling of muscular strength by toning all the body muscles.

26. It counteracts feelings of fatigue.

27. It augments a chemical action which increases the potential of body cells.

28. It causes muscles to move vital fluids throughout the body which in turn lessens the work done by the heart.

29. It has a stabilizing effect on blood pressure and

normalizes it.

30. It releases the flow of endorphins which are the body's own tranquilizers.

31. It has a hardening and strengthening effect on bones of the entire skeletal system.

32. It provides a reserve of body strength and physical efficiency.

33. It betters the ratio between high density and low density components of cholesterol which lessens the risk of artery disease and many cancers.

34. It greatly improves mental outlook, optimism, morale and self esteem.

So there you are. With all that walking can do for you and your FMS, you can't help but improve your physical and mental status. The time is now to begin turning your life around. Step number one is to make an appointment with your personal medical advisor and discuss your intentions with him or her. Take this book with you and get his or her input. Let him or her help you to set some realistic goals. And if you can, start walking!

Get Started Exercising With Fibromyalgia

If you have Fibromyalgia, and especially if you have been sedentary, a couch potato, and want to start exercising, it's very important to start slowly. Get direction from your physician and a competent trainer or physical therapist.

Begin with easy, non-stressing stretching exercises and gentle, low-impact activity, such as walking, swimming, or bicycling. Muscle soreness is normal when you are just starting an exercise regimen; however, if you have sharp pain, stop and call your physician or trainer. You don't want to overwork or injure your muscles, joints, or tendons.

There are no particular exercises to avoid if you have Fibromyalgia as long as they don't do injury. Aerobic exercise such as running, jogging, weight training, water exercise, and flexibility exercises can all help. Recreational activities like golf, tennis, hiking, are usually also healthful.

Take note that If you have other medical problems or if you're planning more than a moderate-intensity exercise program, discuss your plan with your physician before you start.

Chapter 8

Psychological and Behavioral Therapies

Cognitive behavioral therapy (CBT) and related psychological behavioral therapies are treatments, which have shown to be quite effective in many cases of FMS. Following are some coping strategies you may want to use to help yourself to live a better life with Fibromyalgia:

Minimize the stress in your life. It is generally agreed that stress plays an important role in triggering Fibromyalgia symptoms. Many, if not most people with FMS tell of feeling anxious, nervous, and panicked around the time when Fibromyalgia symptoms flare. When Fibromyalgia patients reduce the stress in their lives, they also tend to experience a reduction in depression, anxiety, sleep disorders, and their chronic fatigue. Sleep becomes more restful and their minds and bodies can relax. They feel more in control, so the symptoms that were once immobilizing subside, and their quality of life improves. *Psychological counseling* may be helpful in learning how to reduce you stress levels. *Relaxing CDs* are a tool that patients often find helpful in reducing stress. Some patients have found *hypnosis* helpful for stress reduction.

Learn to remove yourself emotionally from your stressful situations. People often magnify their problems, making them seemingly far greater than really they are. The stress is usually triggered by perception. When you imagine something as a crisis situation, when in reality it isn't, your body reacts as if you are in jeopardy. Learn to temper your emotions as problems arise throughout your day. Instead of seeing every bad event as a crisis, learn to view life's interruptions as a tolerable inconvenience that you can easily handle.

Make job site modifications. To keep working you must stay mentally and physically able to handle your job responsibilities. To avoid job stress and anxiety, you may need to allow more time during the day to get your tasks done. Talk to your employer and try to work out a flexible schedule that allows you to come in later and leave later. Discuss if you can work at home so you can get more rest or take a nap at lunchtime to boost your energy. Budget your time, and learn to limit your outside commitments on work days.

Work to improve communication skills. Free and open communication is important with any chronic condition, Fibromyalgia included. Candid and honest communication helps decrease conflict between you and your spouse, family, friends, and co-workers. Remember that FMS is a little understood disease, so it is vital you help others understand your problems and needs. This is especially vital when you are having unending pain and fatigue. These distractions can hinder productive communication. Remember, if you feel overwhelmed with the stress of Fibromyalgia, psychological counseling can help you to develop better appropriate and functional communication strategies to deal with your disease and others in your life.

Learn to say "no." Failing to set personal limits to too many demands may overburden and over stress you. To help yourself say "no" to a persuasive friend or employer think through the requested situation and what demands it will put on you before you answer. Check your calendar, and consider options and alternatives. Involve others, family members, fellow employees, or friends in the discussion about what to do. The desire to help others is commendable, however, trying to be all things to all people may be exacerbating your symptoms and making you feel resentful, tired, anxious and depressed. It's important at times to take a firm stand, say "no," and mean it.

Keep a daily journal. Writing in a journal daily can become a great tool to help you understand your feelings and your disease. A daily journal may help you to identify events that are associated with the beginning of your Fibromyalgia symptoms and flares. That can help you understand how and when symptoms start, and perhaps avoid your triggers. Keeping a journal can also assist you in tracking your muscle pain and fatigue and in identifying what may cause them. Months later, you might look back on a journal entry and recognize a pattern that identifies a relationship between your increased FMS symptoms and evident lifestyle triggers.

Soak in a warm bath. Relaxing in a warm bath, standing under a warm shower, soaking in a hot tub, or resting in sauna can benefit you in two ways; it will help you to relax your tense muscles, reducing your pain, and help you move more easily, and secondly, the moist heat may raise levels of endorphins and decrease levels of stress hormones. Furthermore, a warm bath before bedtime can help sleep be more deep and restful. Heat pack to specific tense or painful areas can also be quite soothing and helpful. Always be cautious that your heat is not so hot as to burn you.

Exercise regularly. We've already covered the benefits of a regular exercise program. Arthritis Foundation emphasizes that exercising regularly is important to ease symptoms of Fibromyalgia. Because of the pain, stiffness, and ongoing fatigue, felt by people with FMS, many patients have become physically unfit. Aerobic or conditioning exercises such as walking, swimming, and biking have both analgesic and antidepressant effects, and can help enhance your sense of well-being and sense of being in control.

Reduce your caffeine intake. Much as people love their coffee or caffeinated soft drinks, caffeine is one of the few food products that may induce a strong stress reaction. Too much caffeine can greatly increase nervousness, anxiety, and especially insomnia. You should limit the amount of caffeine you ingest as you try to de-stress your life. Also remember tea and chocolate also contain caffeine as do other beverages.

Use mind and body relaxation tools and methods. There are numerous relaxation techniques, tools, and methods you can use to ease your daily tension, anxiety, depression, and pain. You can learn relaxation with guided imagery, visualization, meditation, progressive muscle relaxation, deep abdominal breathing, self-hypnosis, and biofeedback. When you meditate and experience the relaxation reaction, your body goes into a calmer, more stress free, and peaceful mood. Electrical brain wave studies show that when you step back from problems and use mind/body methods to relax, you produce brain waves consistent with serenity and happiness. Talking to a counselor about ways to **change negative to positive self-talk** so you can become more optimistic about yourself and your illness can be extremely helpful.

Evaluate your sleep environment. Make sure your body and sleep environment are totally prepared for restful slumber. You can't sleep well if there is excessive light in your room or if a TV is ear-piercing in another room. Your sleeping quarters should be quiet, dark, and cool. Use earplugs if you are sensitive to noise, and wear an eye mask to block ambient light. Eliminate caffeine within five hours before sleep, and exercise regularly, though not within three hours before bedtime. Sometimes a snack that's high in carbohydrates will help induce sleep because it boosts levels of serotonin in your body as does warmed milk. Serotonin is a chemical neurotransmitter that helps regulate mood, appetite, and sleep.

Join a Fibromyalgia support group. Support groups are geared toward meeting the needs of people with FMS. Support groups are often educational, and are not usually psychotherapy groups. They are designed to provide patients and their families with a safe and accepting environment where they can vent their frustrations, share their personal stories, and receive comfort and encouragement from others. It can be very beneficial to share experiences with other FMS patients and their families. A support group can be a source for knowledge about FMS and you may learn valuable techniques from other patients on how to improve your own lifestyle. Ask your physician for group recommendations or check with the Arthritis Foundation for support groups in your area.

Above all make time for yourself every day. Work for an overall lifestyle balance and make yourself numero uno. You have to put your health needs ahead of some of the needs of others, and make time to do the things you want to do as well as the things you need to do. People with Fibromyalgia are faced with special demands that other people do not have, and the tasks of coping with pain and fatigue each day makes it essential to keep your priorities in order so you have the energy and wherewithal to reach your every day goals.

Chapter 9

The Long-Term Outlook for People With Fibromyalgia

As with many chronic conditions, patients with Fibromyalgia tend to have good days and bad. With proper FMS treatment, which should include regular exercise and physician guidance, most people have decent symptom relief. However, characteristically the pain will come back from time to time, especially when life becomes stressful. Over time, most patients will learn what helps them work through these painful episodes and how to help prevent them. Every patient is different, but with time you'll discover what activities and lifestyle changes will work for you. With the multitude of treatment options available to FMS patients today, there has never been a more favorable prognosis for Fibromyalgia sufferers.

There is no doubt that FMS patients who continue to stay active physically as well as socially, despite their pain, end up doing the best.

Coping with Fibromyalgia is becoming easier than ever before because of a multifaceted treatment approaches that involve medications and lifestyle strategies, the prospects for people with Fibromyalgia much better than ever before.

Learning how to self-manage FMS symptoms with exercise and other lifestyle habits is fundamental to improving your mood, improve your sleep, and get relief from your pain. Furthermore, many people with Fibromyalgia are often caring for others, either by parenting or care giving for an older loved one. Even more FMS patients hold down jobs with responsibilities they can't ignore. Yet they allow too little time to take care of their own health and well being needs.

The limitations of Fibromyalgia can be lessened if you understand the facts of the disease. One of the most important things you can do is learn all you can about the disease and how it is treated. Seek the latest information on FMS and the lifestyle habits that can ease your burden. Get answers to your questions from your physician, physical therapists, trainers, pharmacists, support groups, and other patients; then take proactive steps to focus on your health. Seek support wherever you can. Increased support will help get your life and priorities in order.

Again, the tips for coping with Fibromyalgia, often more important than medication:

❖ **Realize you are not alone.** About 5 million Americans suffer from the pain and fatigue of FMS. There is no "pill" to cure your disease or symptoms, however, there are ways of managing them so they don't disrupt your busy life as to as great an extent.

❖ **Minimize stress in your life**

❖ **Remove yourself emotionally from**

stressful situations

❖ Make job site modifications

❖ Work to improve communication skills

❖ Learn to say "no

❖ Keep a daily journal

❖ Soak in a warm bath

❖ Exercise regularly

❖ Eliminate or reduce caffeine intake

❖ Use mind and body tools and methods for relaxation

❖ Evaluate your sleep hygiene

❖ Consider joining a fibromyalgia support group

❖ Make time for yourself each day

The costs of Fibromyalgia to patients and families

Patients with Fibromyalgia and their families usually have higher health care utilization and costs. Of almost 20,000 Humana members enrolled in Medicare Advantage and commercial plans the compared costs and medical utilizations it was found that persons with Fibromyalgia used twice as much pain-related medication as those without FMS. Also, the use of medications and medical necessities increased markedly across many measures once a FMS diagnosis was made.

Although FMS is neither degenerative nor fatal, the chronic pain of Fibromyalgia is chronic, pervasive, and persistent, and most Fibromyalgia patients report that their symptoms do not go away over time. Though the treatment options for FMS patients have markedly increased, so has the cost of treatment, both because there are numerous new treatment options and the fact that the economy has driven up the heavy cost of medical care.

Chapter 9

Stressed Or Distressed?
Reprioritize!

We all suffer from all kinds of stresses, and these stresses, whatever they may be, when frustrating enough can lead to lots of other physical illnesses.

If there is one remarkable similarity among healthy and happy folks it's the lack of **distress** and more important, **anger**, in their lives. We emphasize the word "distress." Distress, not stress, is the problem. Distress and its resultant **anger** is what makes us sick and kills too many of us.

Stress can actually be good for it is what motivates us to get things done. It pushes us off dead center ... makes us climb out of ruts. It's when we can't do anything about our stress that we get **distressed** and angry. It is the distress and anger and their accompanying frustrations, irritations, feelings of futility, failure and disappointment, causing even deeper anger that destroys out health and shortens our lives.

For most of us "distress and anger" are the most difficult aspects of our lifestyles to eliminate or change. This is especially so if we also have a low self-esteem because we don't like how we function or feel. Too many of us have set goals that are too demanding, unrealistic or plain impossible for ourselves. For some crazy reason we insist on "keeping up with Jones," or worse, "we want to be Jones!" And when we feel we are failures because we can't even control our pain or our everyday lives, and drill into ourselves our shortcomings, then our accomplishments are all the more important to us.

In our fantasy life we want to be seen as heroes and giants in our fields of work. We want to be financial successes beyond anyone's dreams. We imagine lofty goals to compensate for our physical shortcomings. In short we want to be envied rather than be pitied or scorned. **We want to be healthy!**

Fortunately, as we get older, most of us tend to mellow out a bit and distress and anger become a little less a factor in our lives. Furthermore, when life threatening illness comes along, it seems to help us put aside some of the crazy goals that have caused us so much distress in our lives. Brushes with severe illness and crises tend to help us reprioritize our lives and values.

Hopefully, this chapter will help you to do just that; **reprioritize your life and values before they cause the distress and anger** that bring on life threatening illnesses. You must learn to let distress and anger play a very minimal role during your long, active and healthy, happy future.

The first distress you must rid yourself of is that caused by the thought that unless you are completely rid of your Fibromyalgia you aren't worth anything. Decide to minimize the effects of your symptoms and become fit as you possibly can. **Positive self-talk!** Develop a scheduled exercise program, and scheduled sleep times. Get good nutritional advice from your health advisors and live by it. Get counseling where and when you need it.

Next, reconsider what is really important to you.

Reprioritize your life and try to eliminate some of the demands you've put on yourself. Most of us have too much food on our tables ... and it always seems to be the wrong kind. Our homes are much more than adequate often with rooms we hardly use. Our clothing is usually abundantly hung in closets and we try to accumulate the latest gadgets and possessions, most of which end up hardly if ever used. So if we're so much better off, why are we so "distressed and angry?"

Perhaps it's those *"cravings!"*

Now we're certainly not suggesting we give up all our material and modern conveniences; far from it. We have nothing against the "good life." But let's reexamine and make sure what we "crave" is really "good," really what we want. Let's make sure the price we pay with "distress" isn't too high.

For example, in our society, most of us need a car. Our pace and distances are too great for us to rely on walking from appointment to appointment. We can buy a car for around $20,000 or less that will usually get us where we want to go with reasonable reliability and comfort. We can buy a $190,000 car and it will usually get us there with reasonable reliability and comfort ... considerable more comfort perhaps ... but probably not $170,000 more comfort. Ah, but the prestige; that may be worth $170,000 to some of us. If we can afford it, the luxury car may be a source of joy and happiness we consider worthwhile. That's where the "good life" may indeed be "good" for you. Are the things we crave, worth the worry and distress, and the aggravated symptoms they cause worth longing?

But, if putting out that extra money, effort, work, and worry causes too much sacrifice, hardship, sleeplessness, and a heap of "distress," that "good life" isn't good for you.

It just can't be worth it. If it harms your health, flares your Fibromyalgia, rethink your priorities and values. Set a more realistic goal.

Now is the best time for you to really reprioritize your life. Take a realistic inventory of your values. Is being at the top of your profession as important to you now as it once might have been? Is being the richest guy in the hospital or cemetery really what you want out of life? Are you going to be able to enjoy all your material possessions, or would you be better off with a few less "things" and a lot more "time" to enjoy your life and family, friends and loved ones?"

STRESS vs. DISTRESS

Stress as we use it in this book means a physical or mental tension, uneasiness, an irritation, a pull, tug or force to bring about a change in the status quo. It does not infer pain, grief, suffering, strain, and frustration. These characteristics we delegate to "distress."

We use stress as that good restlessness that provokes you to some action. Distress, on the other hand, is worry, frustration agony, pain, etc., resulting when your actions don't work out as desired. That brings on "anger" and anger is what will do you in, especially if the anger is directed toward yourself. Anger is what will cause you hypertension, ulcers, heart attacks, strokes, Fibromyalgia flares, and a host of other dread diseases.

If you were a great big world-class weight lifter and had a shot at the Olympics, no doubt you would come under considerable stress prior to the tryouts. If that stress made you work out harder, resulting in top fitness, improving your chances, it would be good. If you felt no stress prior to the tryouts you probably wouldn't push yourself to attain peak conditioning. On the day of the tryouts you would probably feel the greatest stress, which would get your adrenalin flowing and add considerably to your success. After the match you would be elated and happy if you placed. All that stress of the previous weeks and months would have benefited you.

If on the other hand, you lost ... didn't place, there would probably be considerable frustration, pain, "the agony of defeat," ... *distress* and its accompanying depression, and **anger!** If you didn't have a mechanism to cope with your distress and anger it could lead to depression, anxiety, feelings of failure and eventually any number of physical and mental ailments. You might even be so frustrated you'd stop working out and that would be real bad.

Stresses remain beneficial as long as they provoke positive action. Once you let them turn to negative action or inaction or become worrisome and self-depreciating, you've got distress. That's what happens with most chronic illnesses, failure, frustration, inaction, self-depreciation, and self directed anger. If your Fibromyalgia is turned into positive stress, you will be coping with your distress, turning it back into positive action. You might decide to change your tack and get into good nutrition and start an exercise walking program, work to improve your sleep habits, and continuously work harder to improve your health situation. All these would be positive reactions to potential distress, defusing it by turning it into other motivating stresses. *The way to cope with distress is to "turn your lemons into lemonade!"*

When you have a setback, don't fret, and stew about it. That does no good. Start with analytical self-talk and then positive suggestion self-talk. Self-destructive reactions are guaranteed to make things worse. Turn your energies into another direction and if need be, return to your problem at a later time when you can face it objectively. Exercise is one of the best ways to defuse distress; and you may be surprised at how often a solution to your distress will come to you, spontaneously, while your attention is diverted to more pleasant activities.

If your life is constantly filled with distress and anger, it is time to take a full accounting of your situation. This may require the help of an objective outsider. Not necessarily a professional counselor, but a trusted friend, a spouse, fellow employee, clergy, parent or child. However, don't discount a professional if the need is there. Get whatever help you need to realign your life's goals, values and dreams. Remember, nothing is worth the ruination of your health.

Reprioritizing and Realistic Goal Setting

When we first start out in our adult life our priorities might be something like this:

1. Profession or job
2. Money
3. Acquiring property and material goods
4. Family
5. Avocations and recreation
6. Nationality, politics
7. Religion
8. Health

When we get older they may realign themselves more like:

1. Family

2. Health

3. Religion

4. Avocation and recreation

5. Profession or job

6. Money

7. Acquiring property and material goods

8. Nationality, politics

That's quite a change around. Often we are so busy chasing after our goals that we don't even realize they've changed. We must take time out every few years or more often and examine ourselves and adjust our goals to fit our new needs and dreams. If we don't make adjustments we find distress rising in every facet of our lives. Have you ever noticed how well adjusted most of those people are who change professions every few years? We tend to look at them as unstable, lost, irresponsible, and generally unsuccessful. Take another hard look at them. They probably spend a lot more time smiling than you do. Distress is not a big factor in their lives. They adjust to their needs by changing directions, trying new things, making fresh beginnings. They cope well. They are survivors. They aren't anchored to rigid goals and they are usually healthy ... not necessarily problem free ... but healthy and happy!

Spend a few days listing your *real* priorities in their proper order. Don't hesitate to move things around in several different orders. Nothing is etched in stone ...

unless they are tombstones. Let us suggest you place health and recreation high on your list. Both are powerful distress and anger reducers.

Recreation

Recreation deserves a place of its own in the treatment of FMS. Quality recreation time providing the good times for which you live is a must. Quality recreation is one of the best vehicles to strengthen your family relationships, solve your problems, and thus reduce your distress and anger levels. It is a powerful method of reducing hypertension, anxiety, depression, fatigue, and promoting a feeling of well-being. As important as recreation is to your health and healthy outlook, it is too often the last thing FMS patients think about. There is possibly nothing that can take your mind off of your symptoms better than recreation.

Quality recreation is different for each of us ... it is the *avocation* you most enjoy. We emphasize the word "avocation." If you happen to be one of those lucky people who work in a profession or job you truly love more than anything else in the world, you still need some form of recreation. You have to be able to get away to something else. It's what prevents job burnout ... and you can burn out on any job no matter how terrific it may be to you.

Find avocations you can really throw yourself into. Try to become dedicated to them. If golf is your thing take the challenge and work at becoming the best golfer you can be. If painting or sculpture is it for you, you don't have to become another Grandma Moses or Picasso, but work at becoming the best artist you can be. If you can't get hooked enough, seek out other avocations. You can't have too many and eventually one will grab you. Remember, the best distress-reducing avocation is one that takes a lot of concentration, demanding that you get your mind off of everything else, especially your FMS symptoms. It has to be able to push your problems right out of your mind. It has to push its way right into "priority one" while you're engaged in its activities. Thus, an avocation that requires skill development and concentration on detail is all the better. In seeking avocations best suited to you try several activities and continue with those that best turn you on. Perhaps a good place to start is to think about some of the things you wanted to do when you were younger but thought you didn't have the time or finances to pursue.

In addition, when you successfully achieve a proficiency in your avocation it will go a long way toward boasting your self-esteem. If you can't think of a niche for yourself, the following may help:

Exercise... We've already learned that exercise is the best distress reducer. If you can find an avocation which requires vigorous body activity, that's all the better. This activity should not take the place of your walking or major exercise program. It must be in addition to your daily walking or scheduled exercise program. Team sports, tennis, golf, hiking, bodybuilding, swimming and gardening are all activities that fit into this category. Once your walking program has put you into adequate physical condition and your physician gives you the "go ahead," these are good distress reducing avocations.

Travel... A vacation is great to revitalize. The main problem is we can't usually take enough of them. As wonderful as it is to get away for two weeks or longer, frequent long weekends are probably better for us. When we come back from very long vacations the distress caused by all the catching up we need to do may undo all the good our vacation did us. If you only get two weeks vacation, ten working days, you may do better by using them around holiday weekends and getting several four or five day trips a year. If you have a job that requires a lot of travel, consider taking a couple of days at the end of your business trip to save on travel costs and take your spouse along.

Bowling.... Bowlers all over the world will despise me for not placing bowling under exercise, but as an exercise it doesn't build up much of a sweat. However, as a game of skill and a way to get out with people and take your mind off of distressing problems, it has plenty going for it. Bowling is a competitive activity in which you can improve the rest of your life. There are fine points that you can work at which will require complete concentration. You can join a league, adding excitement and good fellowship ... or you can just challenge yourself with constant improvement. One thing you have to watch out for in most bowling alleys is the side stream smoke. More and more bowling alleys are now seeing the benefit of starting smoke-free leagues and making part of their lanes non-smoking. If you can't find one of these more progressive places, suggest to the manager he consider this option.

Music..."Music tames the savage beast!" There may be no truer statement. Perhaps that is why many conductors, composers, and musicians can remain active into their late eighties and nineties. Here we're not suggesting you be only a spectator; you're never too old to take music lessons. Did you ever wish you'd taken up an instrument as a kid? Perhaps you did take lessons but didn't pursue it as far as you'd liked. No better time than the present to remedy that mistake. I know a fifty-eight year old executive who took up the French horn two years ago and has become quite proficient at it. He has also become involved with Barber Shop singing and travels to national and international competitions. Music has become a real top priority in his life and he'll tell you he's never enjoyed life more.

Camping... This is a fun and challenging way to travel and meet new and interesting people. You can back pack in (after your walking program puts you into adequate physical condition) or you can drive to the thousands of campgrounds throughout the world. You can buy or rent a recreational vehicle and have the freedom of a modern day Gypsy. You might try taking a wilderness course to develop some real survival skills. Once you can break the bonds of hotels and motels, the world really becomes yours with limitless frontiers to explore. There is no better way to bond or re-bond with family and friends.

Carpentry... If you are talented with your hands and have a creative tendency, consider carpentry or model building. What can be more satisfying and distress reducing than to see your own creations come to life as you build with woods and tools? This is an avocation in which you will constantly improve and develop new skills. And if woods don't turn you on, perhaps metals will. We know an employee from a large wrecking company who one day started welding together bits and pieces of junk and today is a sculptor of note. His avocation has opened whole new vistas to him as he travels to showings of his "works."

Painting... Water color, oils, acrylics, chalk, crayons, pencils, inks, charcoal, all await you to give them a try. You may never sell a picture, but that isn't the main purpose. There are few activities that can be more absorbing than to dabble in paint, color, form.... You don't have to possess great talent to enjoy art. A few lessons and you'll be able to express yourself surprisingly well on paper or canvas. Art skills can be learned to a point where they become at least self-satisfying and totally absorbing ... and that's the main idea. But don't be surprised if you discover a real hidden talent once you give your creativity a chance to nurture.

Sculpture.... Who didn't enjoy modeling clay as a child? Why not try the adult version. Sculpture, ceramics, origami, welding, carving, paper machete are just a few of the ways for you to create in three dimension.

Reading... No matter what other avocation you may choose, there are times when nothing beats a good book in which to lose yourself. Create time for yourself to get through some of those books you didn't have time for in the past. You might want to join a Great Books group and share your love for literature with new friends and family. And if good books are your passion, you may want to expand into collecting rare books. Also consider doing volunteer work for your local library association.

Writing... As a writers we can tell you first hand, there is no more forgiving art form than writing. Anyone can do it! And just about everyone has said at one time or another, "I'd like to write a book about...." Well, there's no time like the present to get started. Writing will completely absorb your mind. You can't do it and worry about anything else that could be causing you distress. If nothing else, write your family history to hand down to your kids and grandchildren. But if you have the least desire to write something else ... a book, articles, poetry, lyrics, scripts ... have at it! The more you write, the more you'll improve, and the more pleasure you'll get from it.

Gardening...A friend of mine who lives in an apartment with no yard space is one of the most avid gardeners I've ever met. His apartment is a virtual greenhouse. Every windowsill, shelf, and table has potted plants. He has more plants on his floor than most of us have in our gardens. I often wonder what he'd do if he had a yard. The point is that gardening can be a wonderful avocation and anyone can get into it. You can get started with just a few pots and plants or even seeds. Gardening can be scaled to your own space and needs. There is no end to how far you can take this hobby. You can specialize in orchids, roses, cacti, succulents, wild flowers, herbs, vegetables, trees, fruits, shrubs, or you can go for it all. You can even breed your own varieties. Get a little dirt under your nails and give it a fair try.

Farming...If gardening isn't enough of a challenge for you, perhaps you'd like to be a weekend farmer. At first I thought this a little far fetched, but then I was surprised to find that a lot of city folks have a few acres in the country that they own or rent for horses, cattle, turkeys, chickens, rabbits, sheep, goats, pigs, dogs, cats and other critters. Some people grow fruits and vegetables and trees. Some just fish their streams or ponds. If you don't want to raise anything, perhaps just having a weekend home on a few acres will take your mind off of the distressing factors in your life.

Investing... To me investing has always been a distressing activity, but that's probably because I tend to invest more than I can afford to lose. I envy those who know what they are doing and come up winners. The fact is, if investing isn't what you do for a living and you can afford to take the plunge, it can be an excellent avocation. If you are the type who enjoys researching companies, knows the ins and outs of the markets, can afford the gamble, then investing can be a legitimate hobby for you. This is especially true if your investments include coins, stamps, art, antiques...

Entrepreneurship... If you qualify for the investing hobby category, then this is just a step beyond. Just don't get into something that adds to your distress!

Volunteer work.... There is perhaps no more satisfying avocation than volunteer work. Helping others who are less fortunate has its own rewards. It's a way of paying back for our own good fortune and blessings. It can be done in any degree and there is no end to organizations needing your help. Churches, synagogues, mosques, hospitals, service organizations, schools, the Red Cross, the Salvation Army, the Peace Corps, Vista, local and international groups, the Boy and Girl Scouts are but a few who need your help and expertise. Try giving a few hours of yourself a week and see what it does to your distress and anger levels. You are a valuable commodity and resource and you owe it to yourself and your community ... your world ... to share yourself with others.

Hiking... If you are near the woods, mountains, lakes, rivers, the countryside, or anywhere else that lends itself to hiking, then by all means hike. It's an avocation in which you can participate with your spouse, the whole family, grandchildren, and friends. On a hiking day you needn't take your daily walk. Just hike further, longer, a little slower and enjoy it more. Look and listen. Notice the animals and birds, plants and trees. Even insects can be fascinating. Observe nature and try to learn about it. Here's an opportunity to slow down and see things that you've been too busy and in too much of a rush to enjoy in years past.

Teaching.... In all the years you've lived and experienced you've learned a lot more than you realize. You have skills and knowledge that others can and want to learn from. Teaching is one of the most satisfying and fun experiences you can imagine. Check around your local schools and universities. Many have adult continuing education programs that offer any number of courses from ballroom dancing to word processing, bookkeeping, languages, and entrepreneurmanship to writing. You can't have had such an uninteresting life that you don't have something to pass on to others. Look upon is as an obligation to share your expertise with others. And if you really can't find something that you can teach to others, then consider taking some courses and broadening your horizons.

Golf... Golf, like bowling, deserves special mention. It has little aerobic exercise value, but it is a skill activity that constantly challenges one and is an excellent hobby. It takes you out of doors, expands your friendships, is something you can do with friends and acquaintances is mind absorbing, and does help you to stay physically limber. If you can walk the course, all the better. And you're never too old to take it up or play. My mother-in-law in her eighties and after her open-heart surgery still played weekly.

Fishing... Fishing is an international pastime. You can practice this art anywhere in the world. From trolling to fly-casting to deep-sea fishing and spear fishing, it's always a challenge. You can get a workout fishing or you can snooze on the bank of a stream or lake waiting for a strike, but whichever you do, it is a good distress reducing activity. Fishing is a great family avocation or you can sneak off by yourself if solitude is what you need.

Flying... This is a rich man's or woman's hobby, but if you can afford it, flying is an adventure in itself. There is powered aircraft or you can go in for gliding if you live where there are good air currents and thermals. If you're real adventurous you might even go in for ballooning or hang gliding. This is certainly not for everyone, but if it's something you've always wanted to do ... why not now?

Boating... Boating is among the world's most practiced pastimes. You can spend millions on a yacht or just a few hundred bucks on a canoe. I'll never forget the sign I saw on a yacht docked in the Bahamas, "The greatest two days in a boat owner's life are the day he buys his boat ... and the day he sells it!" What the sign didn't tell me was that most boat owners sell their boats only to turn around and buy a bigger one!

Photography... Photography is an activity that works in

combination with almost any other hobby you might choose. With today's amazing and amazingly inexpensive automatic cameras, and digital equipment, almost anyone can be an expert photographer. And with the easy-to-use video cameras you can even be your own movie producer.

Learning... Today there are so many adult education courses offered by public schools, colleges, churches, synagogues, mosques, organizations, museums, galleries and private institutions, you can study almost anything you want. Learning in itself is a wonderful hobby, but more importantly, it can introduce you to many other exciting activities and interests to pursue in the future. The old adage, "you can't teach an old dog new tricks," isn't true. The problem is that too many of us "old dogs" just don't try. Put forth the effort and you can learn anything you want and the more you learn the easier it becomes.

Stamp collecting... This is a hobby you can apply yourself to in all degrees. Perhaps you want to limit yourself to stamps of one type, like sports stamps from all countries, or stamps from all the places you've visited ... or maybe you want to go in for investing in rare stamps. This avocation can be limited to your kitchen table or it can take you all over the world to stamp shows and conventions.

Dancing... Ballroom dancing is making a real comeback these days with competitions and clubs popping up everywhere. Or maybe you just want to be able to "cut a mean rug" once in a while at parties or on nights out. Perhaps you'd like to get into a tap dancing class. Dancing is a very healthy avocation, giving you a good workout while taking your mind off of disturbing factors in your life. Dancing lessons are readily available almost anywhere.

Biking.... If you have good bike paths available to you give it a try. It doesn't take the place of your daily walking, but it makes an excellent additional activity. You should be able to rent a bike to give it a fair trial before investing in your own. Bicycles aren't cheap anymore and the technology has changed considerably since the last time you rolled up your pant leg and took a turn.

Collecting... Collecting anything, stamps, coins, art, antiques, old cars, rare books, whatever strikes your fancy, can be a wonderful avocation. Collecting can take you to all corners of the world, or it can bring the world to you. You'll meet other people with similar interests to yours and you might find yourself owning some real treasures. Most important the study, travel and challenge of collecting will go a long way to reducing the distress of your daily life. Just making the rounds of garage and lard sales or estate sales in your local area can take your mind off of your distresses and FMS.

The above listing is just a scratch in the surface of all the leisure time activities you can get involved in. The most important thing is that you get involved. Don't limit yourself to just one avocation. The more you engage in, the broader your interests will be and the better, more relaxed you'll be for it. Above all, learn to enjoy life. Don't surrender to your FMS. Reprioritize! The things that you've let distress you all of your life probably were never as important as you made them. We create most of our distress ... and we can rid ourselves of distress with just a little effort ... and fun!

Chapter 10

Resources, Organizations And Links

International Association for CFS/ME (IACFS/ME)
27 N. Wacker Drive Suite 416
Chicago, IL 60606
(847) 258-7248
Website: **www.iacfs.net**
A professional organization for physicians and individuals. Annual membership fee is $100.00 for researchers, clinicians, and therapists. For students, patients, and other interested individuals the annual fee is $40.00. Sponsors bi-annual physician/patient conferences on CFS/ME and FMS.

Fibromyalgia Network
PO Box 31750
Tucson, AZ 85751-1750
(800) 853-2929
Website: **www.fmnetnews.com**
Fibromyalgia Network produces the "Fibromyalgia Network Journal," monthly eNews Alerts, and other support and educational materials for an annual membership fee of $28.00. **It maintains referral listings of support groups and health care providers for each state.** *A free information packet is available by writing, calling, or sending a self-addressed stamped envelope (42 cents postage) to FM Network. The packet contains a brochure on FMS/CFS, an order form for Membership, and other educational*

materials available for purchase, including:
Fibromyalgia Network Journal *($28.00)*
Diet and Exercise Supplement *($10.00)*
Relationships Supplement *($9.00)*

Haworth Medical Press
10 Alice Street
Binghamton, NY 13904
(800) 429-6784
Website: www.haworthpress.com
Publisher of three peer-reviewed medical journals relating to MPS/FMS/CFS.
Journal of Musculoskeletal Pain - *$75.00/yr*
Journal of the Chronic Fatigue Syndrome - *$60.00/yr*
Pain and Palliative Care Pharmacotherapy - *$45.00/yr*

Men with Fibromyalgia
The author of this website feels that men have been "quiet too long." This site addresses various issues surrounding men and fibromyalgia. If you are a man with fibromyalgia or have a spouse or male friend with the illness, visit this website. Women always welcome.
Website: www.menwithfibro.com

Massachusetts CFIDS Association
PO Box 690305
Quincy, MA 02269-0305
(617) 471-5559
Website: www.masscfids.org
The **Massachusetts CFIDS Association** *provides information and supportive services to help patients, their families*

and loved ones cope more effectively with CFIDS and FMS.

Fibromyalgia Information Foundation
PO Box 19016
Portland, OR 97280
Website: www.myalgia.com
*Hosts patient conventions and offers excellent videos on exercise,
stretching, and relaxation by* **Sharon Clark, FNP, Ph.D.,** *and*
Robert Bennett, M.D.

Restless Legs Syndrome Foundation, Inc.
1610 14th St NW, Ste 300
Rochester, MN 55901
(877) INFO-RLS
(877) 463-6757
Website: www.rls.org
*The Association publishes the Nightwalkers Newsletter and Medical
Bulletin for $25.00.*

To Your Health, Inc.
17007 E Colony Dr, Ste 107
Fountain Hills, AZ 85268
(800) 801-1406
Website: www.e-tyh.com
*TyH provides a wide variety of mail-order nutritional supplements.
They also publish a quarterly newsletter available for $25.00/yr, with
all the latest information on new supplements.*

Gero-Vita International
4936 Younge St
Toronto, ON M2N 6S3
(800) 406-1314
Website: www.gvi.com

Gero-Vita is an international chain that sells nutritional supplements. Once you place an order, you will automatically receive their full-color magazine which is published monthly.

PUBLICATIONS AND VIDEOS:
FMS Fact Sheet
Prepared by Kristin Thorson, President AFSA
Click here to open Fact Sheet (PDF)
Condensed information on FMS, including demographics, disability studies, research findings, the current status of NIH spending on the condition and more. In PDF format for easy printing, no reprint permission is required for the use and distribution of this document. If you do not have Adobe Acrobat Reader, it is free and can be downloaded by clicking below:
Fibromyalgia Network
Quarterly Journal
(800) 853-2929
This 20+ page quarterly Journal is available from the publisher. The cost is $28.00/yr.For more information visit **www.fmnetnews.com**.

Oregon Fibromyalgia Foundation Exercise DVDs
by Sharon Clark, FNP, Ph.D. and Robert Bennett, M.D.
Three DVDs available: **Balance and Strength, Aerobic Exercises,** *and* **Stretching and Relaxation**. *$30.00 for the first DVD, $22.00 for all others (including postage and handling). Available at:* **www.myalgia.com**.

Headache Help
by Laurence Robbins, M.D. and Susan S. Lang
Published by Houghton Mifflin Company
ISBN: 0-618-04436-1
This book is 288 pages. The cost is $15.00. Available through

online bookstores.

Management of Headache and Headache Medications, Second Edition by Lawrence Robbins, M.D. Published by Springer-Verlag New York, Inc. ISBN: 0-387-98944-7

This book is 296 pages. The cost is $53.95. Available through online bookstores.

Information on the Robbins Headache Clinic is at: www.headachedrugs.com

Fibromyalgia: Up Close and Personal
by Mark J. Pellegrino, M.D.
Published by Anadem Publishing
ISBN: 1-890018-50-3
This book is 424 pages. The cost is $24.50. Available though the OHIO Rehab Center at **(330) 498-9865**.

All About Fibromyalgia
by Daniel J. Wallace, M.D. and Janice Brock Wallace
Published by Oxford University Press
2001 Evans Rd
Cary, NC 27513
(800) 451-7556
This book is 272 pages. The cost is $30.00. For more information visit the publisher's ?website: **www.oup-usa.org**.

Fibromyalgia
by Don L. Goldenberg, M.D.
Published by The Berkley Publishing Group
This book is 256 pages. The cost is $15.95. For more information visit the?publisher's website: **www.penguinputnam.com**.

The Yeast Connection and the Woman

by William G. Crook, M.D.
Wellness Health and Pharmaceuticals
2800 South 18th Street
Birmingham, AL 35209
(800) 227-2627
This book is 731 pages. The cost is $17.95. For more information please contact the publisher.

CANADIAN REFERENCES:
FM-CFS Canada
For support groups and help throughout Canada, visit the FM-CFS Canada. Resources in English and French.
Website: www.fm-cfs.ca

MEFM
The Myalgic Encephalomyelitis and
Fibromyalgia Societies of BC
Box 462, 916 West Broadway Ave
Vancouver, BC V5Z 1K7
Canada
(604) 878-7707
Website: www.mefm.bc.ca
Publishes a quarterly newsletter for an annual membership fee of $15.00. Offers support group listings and other educational materials for sale or rent.

OTHER RESOURCES:
The CDC's 1994 CFS criteria article from Annuals of Internal Medicine can be downloaded at:
http://www.cdc.gov/cfs/cfsdefinition.htm.
The Journal of SLEEP has a home page in which you may download interesting scientific abstracts pertaining to sleep research. Their site is: **www.journalsleep.org**

Headache Help - a website developed by Lawrence Robbins, M.D., a neurologist who runs a headache clinic in Illinois and who also suffers with chronic, daily headache pain. It is devoted to helping patients treat their headaches and to keep patients/physicians current on the latest remedies for migraine and tension-type headaches. This website is located at: **www.headachedrugs.com**
The following are web sites that provide information on chronic pain treatments and prescription guidelines:
www.AmPainSoc.org
www.Partnersagainstpain.com
www.fsmb.org
www.painpolicy.wisc.edu (The Pain and Policy Studies Group site hosted by University of Wisconsin

APPENDIX I

ARTHRITIS RELATED STATISTICS

PREVALENCE OF ARTHRITIS

An estimated 46 million adults in the United States reported being told by a doctor that they have some form of arthritis, rheumatoid arthritis, gout, lupus, or fibromyalgia. One in five (over 21%) adults in the United States report having doctor diagnosed arthritis. In 2003–2005, 50% of adults 65 years and over reported an arthritis diagnosis. By 2030, an estimated 67 million of Americans aged 18 years or older are projected to have doctor-diagnosed arthritis. An estimated 294,000 children under age 18 have some form of arthritis or rheumatic condition; this represents approximately one in every 250 children.

Prevalence of Specific Types of Arthritis

The most common form of arthritis is osteoarthritis. Other common rheumatic conditions include gout, fibromyalgia and rheumatoid arthritis. An estimated 21 million adults have osteoarthritis. An estimated 2.1 million adults are affected by rheumatoid arthritis. An estimated 5.1 million adults report having a doctor diagnosis of gout. An estimated 3.7 million adults have fibromyalgia.

Prevalence of Arthritis by Age/Race/Gender

Of persons aged 18–44, 7.9% (8.7 million) report doctor-diagnosed arthritis. Of persons aged 45–64, 29.3% (20.5 million) report doctor-diagnosed arthritis. Of persons aged 65+, 50.0% (17.2 million) report doctor-diagnosed arthritis, 28.3 million women and 18.1 million men report doctor-diagnosed arthritis, 3.1 million Hispanic adults report doctor-diagnosed arthritis, 4.6 million Non-Hispanic Blacks report doctor-diagnosed arthritis. An estimated 294,000 children under age 18 have some form of arthritis or rheumatic condition; this represents approximately one in every 250 children.

Overweight/Obesity and Arthritis (adult aged 18)

People who are overweight or obese report more doctor-diagnosed arthritis than thinner people, 16% of under/normal weight adults report doctor-diagnosed arthritis, 21.7% of overweight and 30.6% among obese Americans report doctor-diagnosed arthritis, 66% of adults with doctor-diagnosed arthritis, are overweight or obese (compared with 53% of adults without doctor-diagnosed arthritis). Weight loss of as little as 11 pounds reduces the risk of developing knee osteoarthritis among women by 50%.

Physical Activity and Arthritis

Almost 44% of adults with doctor-diagnosed arthritis report no leisure time physical activity compared with 36% of adults without arthritis. Among older adults with knee osteoarthritis, engaging in moderate physical activity at least 3 times per week can reduce the risk of arthritis-related disability by 47%.

Disability/Limitations and Arthritis

State-specific prevalence estimates of arthritis-attributable work limitation show a high impact of arthritis on working-age (18-64 years) adults in all U.S. states, ranging from a low of 3.4% to a high of 15% of adults with arthritis in this age group. Approximately 5% of ALL U.S. adults between the ages of 18 and 64 in this age group are affected by arthritis-attributable work limitation. Approximately 1 in 3 people with arthritis in this age group report arthritis-attributable work limitation Arthritis and other rheumatic conditions are a leading cause of disability in the United States. Among all civilian, non-institutionalized U.S. adults 8.8% (19 million) report both doctor-diagnosed and arthritis attributable "activity limitations." Nearly 41% of adults with doctor-diagnosed arthritis report arthritis-attributable activity limitations. Among adults with doctor-diagnosed arthritis, many report significant limitations in vital activities such as:

❖ walking 1/4 mile—6 million
❖ stooping/bending/kneeling—7.8 million
❖ climbing stairs—4.8 million
❖ social activities such as church and family gatherings—2.1 million

Among all civilian, non-institutionalized U.S. adults, aged 18-64, 4.8% (8.2 million) report both doctor diagnosed arthritis and arthritis-attributable work limitations, 30.6% of adults aged 18-64 with doctor-diagnosed arthritis report an arthritis-attributable work limitation.

Health Related Quality of Life (HRQOL) and Arthritis

Persons with doctor-diagnosed arthritis have significantly worse HRQOL than those without arthritis. People with doctor-diagnosed report more than twice as many unhealthy days and three times as many days with activity limitations in the past month than those without arthritis.

Arthritis Healthcare Utilization
Hospitalizations

In 1997, there were an estimated 744,000 hospitalizations with a principal diagnosis of arthritis (3% of all hospitalizations).

Outpatient Care

There were 36.5 million ambulatory care visits for arthritis and other rheumatic conditions in 1997, or nearly 4% of all ambulatory care visits that year.

Arthritis-Related Mortality

From 1979-1998, the annual number of arthritis and other related rheumatic conditions (AORC) deaths rose from 5,537 to 9,367. Three categories of AORC account for almost 80% of deaths: diffuse connective tissue diseases (34%), other specified rheumatic conditions (23%), and rheumatoid arthritis (22%). In 1979, the crude death rate from AORC was 2.46 per 100,000 populations. In 1998, it was 3.48 per 100,000 population; rates age-standardized to the year 2000 population were 2.75 and

3.51, respectively.

Arthritis Costs

In 2003, the total cost attributed to arthritis and other rheumatic conditions in the United States was 128 billion dollars, up from 86.2 billion dollars in 1997. Medical expenditures (direct costs) for arthritis and other rheumatic conditions in 2003 were 80.8 billion dollars, up from 51.1 billion in 1997. Earnings losses (indirect costs) for arthritis and other rheumatic conditions in 2003 were 47 billion dollars, up from 35.1 billion in 1997.

Mental/Emotional Health and Arthritis

Arthritis is strongly associated with major depression (attributable risk of 18.1%), probably through its role in creating functional limitation.

Total Joint Replacements in Arthritis

In 2003, there were 418,000 total knee replacements performed, primarily for arthritis.

APPENDIX II
QUIT SMOKING NOW

Dr. Seiden believes in prevention being more important than the cure, therefore, the detrimental side effects of smoking are well documented and many times, smoking increases Arthritis symptoms and suffering.

Dr. Seiden has written and published a full course on how to Quit Smoking Now and he gives this away to anyone who has a desire to quit or simply wants some more information.

Please   visit BoomerBookSeries.com/QuitSmokingNow.php   and download your free 66 page e-book to Quit Smoking Now!

RECOMMENDED READING

THE ARTHRITIS HELPBOOK BY KATE LORIG & JAMES FRIES
ISBN: 0738210706

THE ANTI-INFLAMMATION DIET AND RECIPE BOOK, PROTECT YOURSELF AND YOUR FAMILY FROM HEART DISEASE, ARTHRITIS, DIABETES, ALLERGIES AND MORE BY N.D. JESSICA K. BLACK
ISBN: 0897934857

THE CLEVELAND CLINIC GUIDE TO ARTHRITIS BY MD JOHN D. CLOUGH
ISBN: 1427799563

ARTHRITIS: THE CURE - THE LAST BOOK YOU'LL EVER NEED ON ARTHRITIS BY MD GEORGE TILDEN
ISBN: 1441465766

COPING WITH ARTHRITIS - BY MD OTHNIEL SEIDEN
ISBN: 0-9844838-6-1 (ALSO AVAILABLE IN KINDLE)

About The Author(s)

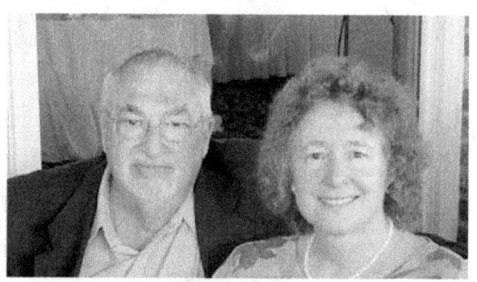

Othniel J. Seiden, M.D.
Jane L. Bilett, Ph.D.

The human animal is intended to be active throughout life and Arthritis, in its many forms has become the *number one debilitating disease* interfering with our mobility and continued function.

Jane L. Bilett, PhD has practiced Clinical Psychology for over 30 years and Othniel J. Seiden, MD medicine for well over 40 years. In addition, Othniel has experienced the disease from the patient's point of view having had two hip replacements.

Together, Jane and Othniel have helped hundreds of individuals to cope with these handicapping diseases. To achieve the best possible mobility and active life through the senior years requires both prevention and cure of these diseases. With their cumulative experience dealing with the psychological and medical aspects of arthritis, they are most qualified to help you retain the best life quality you can hope for!

More From Othniel

Health

5 HTP The Serotonin Connection:
*The Natural Supplement that helps
you be in control of your mind and body!*
ISBN: 1519148445
5-HTP and Depression Management:
Available in Kindle Only
5HTP and Memory Loss Management with:
Available in Kindle Only
5 HTP PMS and Menopause:
Available in Kindle Only
Coping with Arthritis:
ISBN: 151941353X
Coping with BPH:
*Benign Prostatic Hypertrophy
Male, over 45, you probably have it!*
Available in Kindle Only
Coping with Colorectal Cancer:
*Prevention and Cure of theSecond Leading
Cause of Cancer Deaths*
Available in Kindle Only
Coping with Fibromyalgia:
It's not in your head, it's a disease!
ISBN: 1519438311

Coping with Prostate Cancer:
Prevention and Cure
of Man's Most Common Cancer
ISBN: 1519438737

Heart of a Woman:
Prevetion and Cure of the #1 Killer in Women
ISBN: 1519441533

Heavy and Healthy:
Forget Your Weight and Get Fit!
ISBN: 1519495412

Quit Smoking Now!:
The Program to Help You
Quit Smoking Now and Forever!
ISBN: 1519495781

Sharpening the Aging Mind:
Methods, Tricks & Tips to
Keep Your Mind Super Sharp
ISBN: 1519496028

Sleep Disorders Management:
Available in Kindle Only

The Second half begins at 50:
Your Longevity Handbook
ISBN: 1519496389

Walk!:
Walk Your Way to Great Health & Long Life
Available in Kindle Only

Weight & Appetite Management:
Available in Kindle Only

Relationships:

Adultery Case Histories:
> *Why People Cheat on Their Partners*
> **Available in Kindle Only**

Communing with the Dead:
> *Death Needn't Part You*
> **ISBN: 1519190085**

Foreplay:
> *The True Focus of Great Sex*
> **ISBN: 1519440979**

Sex in the Golden Years:
> *The Best Sex Ever, Stay Sexually Active for Life*
> **ISBN: 1519495927**

The Big O:
> *Male & Female Multiple Orgasms*
> **ISBN: 1519496109**

The Hospice Experience:
> *Making Your Most Important Final Decision*
> **ISBN: 1519496281**

When Your Spouse Dies:
> *A widow's & widower's handbook*
> **ISBN: 151949646X**

Jewish Fiction

Padre Pio:
> *The Capuchin – the life of Padre Pio -*
> *St. Pio of Pietrelcina*
> *Sex, Horror & Violence vs. Unyielding Faith!*
> **ISBN: 1519495684**

Seed of Avraham:
>*A 4000 Year History of the Jewish Family...*
>>>**ISBN: 1519495811**

Shtetl:
>>*The Story of a Life No More...*
>>*As told from the hereafter*
>>>**ISBN: 1519496036**

The Cartographer:
>>>*1492*
>>>**ISBN: 151949615X**

The Condemned Voyage:
>>*The S.S. St. Louis - 1939*
>>>**Available in Kindle Only**

The Crusades:
>*The Jewish World of the 12th Century*
>>>**Available in Kindle Only**

The Death of Berlin:
>*A Story of Hollocaust Survival and Revenge*
>>>**Available in Kindle Only**

The Remnant:
>>*The Jewish Resistance in WWII*
>>>**ISBN: 1519496346**

The Uprising of Babi Yar:
>>*The Syrets Deathcamp*
>>>**Available in Kindle Only**

Miscellaneous

Guaranteed Routes to Success for Writers:
>*A Road Map Through Today's*
>*Dramatic Changes in Publishing*
>>>**Available in Kindle Only**

Joy of Volunteering:
Working and Surviving in Developing Countries
ISBN: 1519495587

So You Want to Write a Book:
ISBN: 1519496079

If you found

Coping with Fibromyalgia

helpful & useful

Please leave a review on
Amazon.com

Also available in Kindle